The Midwifery Test Book

The Midwifery Test Book

**Edited by Helen Wightman
and Robina Aslam**

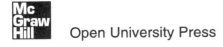
Open University Press

Open University Press
McGraw-Hill Education
McGraw-Hill House
Shoppenhangers Road
Maidenhead
Berkshire
England
SL6 2QL

email: enquiries@openup.co.uk
world wide web: www.openup.co.uk

and Two Penn Plaza, New York, NY 10121–2289, USA

First published 2012

A catalogue record of this book is available from the British Library

ISBN-13: 978-0-33-524479-9 (pb)
ISBN-10: 0-33-524479-3 (pb)
eISBN: 978-0-33-524480-5

Library of Congress Cataloging-in-Publication Data
CIP data applied for

Illustrations by Gary Holmes
Typesetting and e-book compilations by
RefineCatch Limited, Bungay, Suffolk
Printed and bound by CPI Group (UK) Ltd, Croydon, CR0 4YY

The McGraw·Hill Companies

Contents

Foreword

I am delighted to have the opportunity to provide a foreword for a new and extremely valuable addition to the resources available to students of midwifery and those who support their education. This text, edited by two experienced midwife educators, offers a range of approaches through which midwifery students and those facilitating them can assess students' developing knowledge and understanding and application of knowledge to practice.

This book can be used in a range of ways: by midwifery students studying alone, as an additional means of testing understanding of both physiological and pathological aspects of midwifery. It would identify areas where tutorial support might be helpful or where a midwifery educator would be able to signpost the student to additional learning opportunities or resources. It could be used at different times in students' training, when concepts are first taught to test understanding, consolidate knowledge or used to support revision prior to summative assessments.

In addition to testing knowledge of anatomy and physiology, its potential to test abilities in care planning uses real-life clinical situations that midwives will encounter regularly in their practice. Other clinical conditions occur less frequently but have potentially serious sequelae and it is important that midwives are also able to identify and respond to these at the point of registration. Additional particularly notable features of *The Midwifery Test Book* are the sections related to pharmacology and medicines administration and numeracy. These are core competencies that midwives must be able to practise safely and additional opportunities for revision are particularly welcome.

Mentors make an essential contribution to the education and assessment of midwifery students and in enabling a skilled workforce. This text is also a resource for them when working clinically with students and the contents are available to reinforce learning.

Whilst midwives' professional responsibilities and the scope of practice may vary between countries, the text has value for pre-registration midwifery students in a range of settings, offering a means of testing core elements of midwifery knowledge.

This text also offers a valuable resource for experienced midwives who are embarking on a career in education as it models a range of approaches to question formulation, including multiple choice questions, short answers, true/false statements and where required, presents model answers.

Finally, whilst focussed on pre-registration students, many midwives progress to further study to advance the breadth and depth of their knowledge. In such situations, an efficient method is needed that will identify areas where knowledge may need to be refreshed before further learning takes place. This text could support that student-led approach to self-appraisal prior to further professional development.

Helen Spiby
Professor in Midwifery

Contributors

Helen Wightman, RGN, RM, BSc (Hons), MSc, PG Dip, Midwifery Lecturer at the University of Nottingham, UK. Labour Ward Coordinator, NUH Trust, Nottingham. Part Two – Pathophysiology.

Robina Aslam, RGN, RM, ADM, PGCEA, MSc, Midwifery Lecturer at the University of Nottingham, UK. Part Two – Pathophysiology.

Jenny Bailey, RGN, RM, DANS, BN, M Med Sci/Clin Ed, Midwifery Lecturer at the University of Nottingham. Part One – Anatomy and Physiology.

Helen McIntyre, RGN, RM, BSc (Hons), MSc, PG Dip, Midwifery Lecturer at the University of Nottingham. Part One – Anatomy and Physiology.

Preface

This book is intended as a revision aid for students undertaking pre-registration midwifery courses. The aim is to assist students with the revision of anatomy and physiology and pathophysiology related to childbirth through the medium of short questions, true/false statements, multiple choice questions, fill in the blanks questions and labelling of diagrams.

The book is divided into two parts. Part 1 will examine students' knowledge of the normal anatomy and physiology related to childbirth. Part 2 examines students' knowledge regarding the pathophysiology surrounding complications related to childbirth. This revision aid should be used in conjunction with textbooks to develop students' knowledge.

It is acknowledged that learning and understanding is also gained from clinical situations, therefore students should utilise experiences and skills they have gained in practice when answering the questions in this book.

Guide to useful resources

Critical Care in Childbearing for Midwives. Mary Billington and Mandy Stevenson. Blackwell Publishing, 2007.

Ross and Wilson Anatomy and Physiology in Health and Illness (11th edn). Anne Waugh and Alison Grant. Churchill Livingstone, Elsevier, 2010.

Principles of Anatomy and Physiology International Student Version (13th edn). Gerard J. Tortora and Bryan H. Derrickson. John Wiley and Sons, 2011.

The Midwives' Guide to Key Medical Conditions: Pregnancy and Childbirth. Linda Wylie and Helen Bryce. Churchill Livingstone, Elsevier, 2008.

www.unicef.org.uk
Unicef UK website

www.nice.org.uk
National Institute for Health and Clinical Excellence

www.rcog.org.uk
Royal College of Obstetricians and Gynaecologists

www.rcoa.ac.uk
Royal College of Anaesthetists

List of abbreviations

AFE	amniotic fluid embolism		IUGR	intrauterine growth restriction
ARM	artificial rupture of membranes		IV	intravenous
BMI	body mass index		IVI	intravenous infusion
BPM	beats per minute		LAM	lactational amenorrhoea
Ca	calcium		LFT	liver function test
CCT	controlled cord traction		LH	luteinising hormone
CMV	cytomegalovirus		LMWH	low molecular weight heparin
CO_2	carbon dioxide		MAP	mean arterial pressure
CRP	C reactive protein		MEOWS	modified early obstetric warning score
CSF	cerebrospinal fluid			
DNA	deoxyribonucleic acid		MMR	measles, mumps and rubella
DVT	deep vein thrombosis		O_2	oxygen
EAS	external anal sphincter		PE	pulmonary embolus
ECG	electrocardiogram		PGD	patient group directive
FBC	full blood count		pH	reaction of a fluid of a scale form 0–15, to determine acidity or alkalinity
FSH	follicle stimulating hormone			
GBS	group B streptococcus			
HCG	human chorionic gonadotrophin		PoM	Prescription only Medicine
HIV	human immunodeficiency virus		PPH	postpartum haemorrhage
			RNA	ribonucleic acid
IAS	internal anal sphincter		SBAR	Situation, Background, Assessment, Recommendation
IM	intramuscular			
IUFD	intrauterine fetal death		VTE	venous thromboembolic event

Common prefixes, suffixes and word roots

Prefix/suffix/ root	Definition	Example
a-/an	deficiency, lack of	*anuria = decrease or absence of urine production*
-aemia	of the blood	*ischaemia = decreased blood supply*
angio	vessel	*angiogenesis = growth of new vessels*
brady	slow	*bradycardia = slow heart beat*
broncho-	bronchus	*bronchitis = inflammation of the bronchus*
card-	heart	*cardiology = study of the heart*
chole-	bile or gallbladder	*cholecystitis = inflammation of gallbladder*
cyto-	cell	*cytology = study of cells*
derm-	skin	*dermatology = study of the skin*
dys-	difficult	*shoulder dystocia = difficulty with delivery of fetal shoulders at birth*
-ema	swelling	*oedema = abnormal accumulation of tissue/fluid*
entero-	intestine	*enteritis = inflammation of the intestinal tract*
erythro-	red	*erthyropenia = deficiency of red blood cells*
gast-	stomach	*gastritis = inflammation of stomach lining*
-globin	protein	*haemoglobin = iron-containing protein in the blood*
haem-/haemo-	blood	*haemocyte = a blood cell (especially red blood cell)*
-hydr-	water	*rehydrate = replenish body fluids*
hepat-	liver	*hepatitis = inflammation of the liver*
intra-	during	*intrapartum = during labour*
-itis	inflammation	*bronchitis = inflammation of the bronchi*
-kinesia	movement, motion	*bradykinesia = slow movements*
leuco-	white	*leucopenia = deficiency of white blood cells*
lymph-	lymph tissue/vessels	*lymphoedema = fluid retention in the lymphatic system*

-lyso/-lysis	breaking down	*hydrolysis = breaking down molecule with water*
myo-	muscle	*myocardium = cardiac muscle*
nephro-	kidney	*nephritis = inflammation of the kidneys*
neuro-	nerve	*neurology = study of the nerves*
-ology	study of	*dermatology = study of the skin*
-oma	tumour	*lymphoma = tumour of the lymph tissue*
os-/osteo-	bone	*osteology = study of bones*
-penia-	deficiency of	*leucopenia = deficiency of white blood cells*
path-	disease	*pathology = study of disease*
pneumo-	air/lungs	*pneumonitis = inflammation of lung tissue*
tachy-	excessively fast	*tachycardia = excessive heart rate*
tox-	poison	*toxicology = study of poisons*
-uria	urine	*haematuria = blood in the urine*
vaso-	vessel	*vasoconstriction = narrowing of vessels*

Introduction

Welcome to *The Midwifery Test Book*. We hope you will find it an invaluable tool throughout your midwifery course and beyond.

This book is primarily a revision aid dealing with normal physiology and pathophysiology in midwifery practice. It is designed to supplement rather than replace your standard textbook. It will enable you to test yourself as you progress through your studies. There is no need to start reading this book from the beginning – you can select the topics in the order that is most helpful to your learning needs.

The book is divided into two parts. The first deals with normal anatomy and physiology of childbirth. The second deals with complications related to childbirth. Each part begins with a brief introduction and contains chapters dealing with pregnancy, the intrapartum and postnatal periods.

There is a variety of question formats enabling you to assess your knowledge and understanding in different ways. These formats are:

- Multiple choice: identify which of the answers are correct.

- True or false: identify if the statement is true or false.

- Labelling diagrams: identify the different elements on the diagram.

- Fill in the blanks: fill in the blanks to complete the statement.

- Short answers: provide brief explanations or solutions.

- Numeracy questions: basic midwifery practice calculations.

Your particular course programme may not necessarily assess you in the same formats. However, it will be beneficial if you attempt all questions. It is a useful skill to learn how to adapt to different approaches. The core knowledge and understanding you require for your course remain the same however the question is framed.

We refer to useful textbooks and other references, including online resources to support your learning. We include a schedule of common prefixes, suffixes and word roots to help you understand how many of the words we use in midwifery are derived. This will also help you to remember and use them correctly. We supplement this with a detailed glossary and again you can use this to familiarise yourself with appropriate language for discussing areas within your chosen profession with both colleagues and clients.

We hope you enjoy using this book and we wish you all the best in your studies.

Happy self-assessment!

PART 1
Anatomy and physiology

INTRODUCTION

It is essential for student midwives to have knowledge of the anatomy and physiology of the main systems prior to conception occurring. This will provide a foundation to build on when considering changes which occur as a result of pregnancy.

Students are required to have knowledge concerning the expected anatomical and physiological changes which occur in the woman as a result of pregnancy. Although normal, some of these changes have a greater effect than others on the various biological systems. Some of these changes can be clinically observed.

Labour is the culmination of pregnancy. In normal circumstances this would be expected to occur between 37 and 42 weeks of pregnancy. Although a continuous process, it is often divided into three stages, namely first, second and third. The following sets of questions relate to all of these stages. Some of the answers will require application of the anatomy and physiology to midwifery clinical practice.

The puerperium is the period following pregnancy and labour when the woman's body systems return to a non-pregnant state. The physical and psychological wellbeing of the mother and her relationship with the baby are assessed by the midwife and health visitor during this time.

When describing an anatomical structure you are expected to include its situation in the body, its shape and size, and its gross and microstructure. You should also state the blood, nerve and lymphatic systems.

Useful resources

Ross and Wilson Anatomy and Physiology in Health and Illness (11th edition). Anne Waugh and Alison Grant. Churchill Livingstone, Elsevier, 2010.

Principles of Anatomy and Physiology International Student Version (13th edition). Gerard J. Tortora and Bryan H. Derrickson. John Wiley and Sons, 2011.

www.unicef.org.uk

Preconception

1

SHORT ANSWER QUESTIONS

Write short answers to the following:

1 Describe the maturation and development of the Graafian follicle within the menstrual cycle.

2 With reference to the menstrual cycle and associated hormones describe the changes which occur in the endometrium.

3 Describe the preparatory processes the sperm undergoes prior to fertilisation.

4 Identify the physiological rationale for folic acid recommendation prior to pregnancy.

5 An optimal body mass index is recommended prior to pregnancy. How can this be achieved from a balanced diet?

6 Describe the process of spermatogenesis.

7 Describe the process of oogenesis.

8 Describe the implantation of the blastocyst.

9   Identify the differences between oral progesterone only and oral combined contraception in their action on the menstrual cycle.

10   Genetic testing with known parental cystic fibrosis may be offered prior to pregnancy. Describe the inheritance pattern of this autosomal recessive condition for parents who are both carriers of cystic fibrosis.

TRUE OR FALSE?

Are the following statements true or false?

11 The uterus is anterior to the large bowel. T

12 The most fertile time during the menstrual cycle are days 26–28. F

13 The normal preconception dose for folic acid is 400 mcg daily. T

14 The first 14 days of the menstrual cycle is the secretory phase. F

15 Ovulation occurs as a result of a surge in progesterone. F

16 Gonadotrophic releasing hormone (GnRH) is secreted from the hypothalamus. T

17 The wall of the uterus consists of three layers, perimetrium, myometrium and endometrium. T

18 The perimetrium is shed every month as a result of the menstrual cycle. F

19 Sperm are produced in the epididymis. F

20 Gonadotrophic releasing hormone (GnRH) in the male stimulates the release of follicle stimulating hormone. T

MULTIPLE CHOICE

Identify one correct answer for each of the following.

21 Name one of the ligaments that supports the ovaries, uterus and cervix:

   a) cruciate ligament
   b) ligamentum teres
   c) patellar ligament
   d) round ligament

22 Which hormone is involved in the menstrual cycle?

   a) prolactin
   b) progesterone
   c) pepsin
   d) parathyroid hormone

23 Gonadotrophic hormone releasing hormone (GnRH) stimulates the release of which hormone from the following?

   a) progesterone
   b) oestrogen
   c) luteinising hormone
   d) prolactin

24 Capacitation is a process the sperm undergoes prior to fertilisation. This takes how long?

   a) 1 hour
   b) 7 hours
   c) 24 hours
   d) 48 hours

25 Which part of the sperm cell is responsible for penetrating the corona radiate of the secondary oocyte for fertilisation to take place?

   a) neck

   b) flagellum

   c) acrosome

   d) centriole

26 Meiosis is the process of cell division which results in:

   a) diploid number of chromosomes

   b) haploid number of chromosomes

   c) replication of identical cells

   d) no change to the chromosomes

27 Genotype can be described as:

   a) the genetic makeup of an individual

   b) the physical features apparent in an individual

   c) the blood type of an individual

   d) being the same in both parents

28 Which of the following methods of contraception affect the menstrual cycle?

   a) condom

   b) intrauterine contraceptive device

   c) diaphragm

   d) combined oral contraceptive pill

29 The dimensions of the non-pregnant uterus are:

   a) 10 cm × 7.5 cm × 5 cm

   b) 7.5 cm × 5 cm × 2.5 cm

   c) 30 cm × 22.5 cm × 20 cm

   d) 8 cm × 6 cm × 3 cm

30   The following is a function of the uterus:

   a) stores urine prior to voiding

   b) produces hormones regulating the menstrual cycle

   c) prepares the endometrium for implantation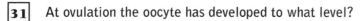

   d) forms the placenta

31   At ovulation the oocyte has developed to what level?

   a) an oogonium

   b) a primary oocyte

   c) a Graafian follicle

   d) a secondary oocyte

32   Describe the correct position of the uterus:

   a) anteverted and anteflexed

   b) retroverted and anteflexed

   c) anteverted and retroflexed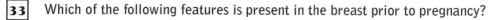

   d) dextrorotated and anteflexed

33   Which of the following features is present in the breast prior to pregnancy?

   a) primary areola

   b) secondary areola

   c) venous engorgement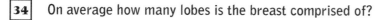

   d) darkening of the areola

34   On average how many lobes is the breast comprised of?

   a) 18

   b) 10

   c) 20

   d) 9

35   Which of the following is the formula for calculating body mass index?

a) height divided by weight

b) weight in kilograms divided by height in metres squared

c) weight divided by height

d) weight squared divided by height

FILL IN THE BLANKS

Fill in the blanks in each statement using the options in the box.

14	human chorionic gonadotrophic
ovarian	genotype
booking	ampulla
growth	secretory (or luteal)
phenotype	proliferative (or follicular)
uterine	

36 Oestrogen stimulates _growth_ of the endometrial lining during the menstrual cycle.

37 Progesterone maintains and further develops the endometrial lining. This is called the _luteal_ phase.

38 Fertilisation generally occurs in the _ampulla_ region of the uterine (fallopian) tubule.

39 Ovulation always occurs _14_ days prior to the menstrual phase.

40 The variation in days of menstrual cycles between different women is dependent on the length in time of the _follicular_ phase.

41 If fertilisation occurs the effects of progesterone in developing the endometrial lining continue as a result of the blastocyst secreting _h c g_ hormone.

42 The genetic material that identifies an individual is called _genotype_.

43 The physical manifestation of genetic material is called _____ *phenotype*

44 During antenatal screening a _____ history is taken. *booking*

45 Blood supply to the cervix is supplied by the _____ and _____ arteries. *ovarian uterine.*

all correct.

LABELLING EXERCISE

Label the following diagrams: the uterus, the menstrual cycle, a sperm, an ovary and genetic inheritance probability pattern.

46–53 Figure 1.1 Uterus

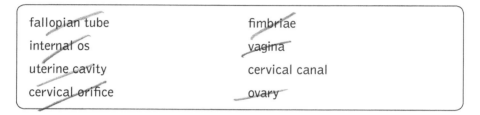

fallopian tube	fimbriae
internal os	vagina
uterine cavity	cervical canal
cervical orifice	ovary

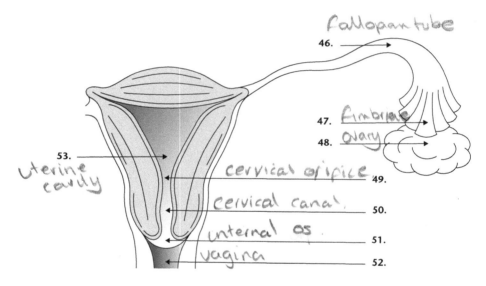

54–58   Figure 1.2 Menstrual cycle – insert the hormones at each stage.

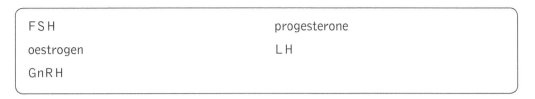

FSH   progesterone

oestrogen   LH

GnRH

Menstrual cycle

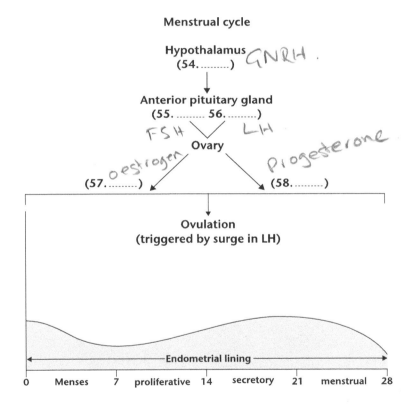

Hypothalamus
(54. ....)   *GNRH .*

↓

Anterior pituitary gland
(55. .... 56. ....)

FSH   *LH*

Ovary

oestrogen   *Progesterone*

(57. ....)   (58. ....)

↓

Ovulation
(triggered by surge in LH)

← Endometrial lining →

0   Menses   7   proliferative   14   secretory   21   menstrual   28

59–63   Figure 1.3 Sperm

mitochondria	centrioles
tail	midpiece
acrosome	nucleus
flagellum	head

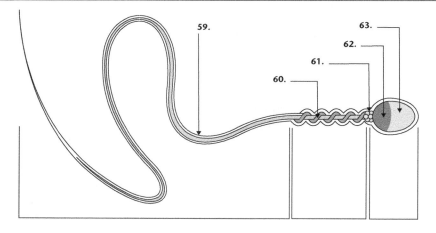

64–82   Figure 1.4 Ovary

blood clot	blood vessels in hilus of ovary
ovarian medulla	germinal epithelium
primary follicle	corona radiata
corpus albicans	granulosa cells
ovarian cortex	ovulation discharges a secondary oocyte
secondary follicle	
corpus luteum	degenerating corpus luteum
zona pellucida	corpus hemorrhagicum (ruptured follicle)
frontal plane	
mature (graafian) follicle	
primordial follicle	
follicular fluid	

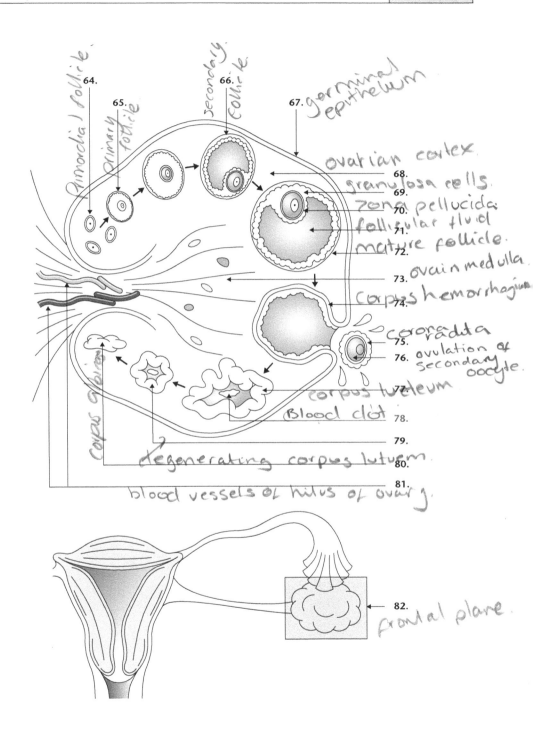

64. primordial follicle.
65. primary follicle
66. secondary follicle.
67. germinal epithelium
68. ovarian cortex.
69. granulosa cells.
70. zona pellucida
71. follicular fluid
72. mature follicle.
73. ovain medulla.
74. corpus hemorrhagium
75. corona radiata
76. ovulation of secondary oocyte.
77. corpus luteum
78. Blood clot
79.
80. degenerating corpus luteum.
81. blood vessels of hilus of ovary.
82. frontal plane.

corpus albicans

83 Complete Figure 1.5 The inheritance pattern for a mother who is blood type O and a father who is blood type A (heterozygous genotype)

Dad \ Mum	-------	-------
-------	-------	-------
-------	-------	-------

ANSWERS

SHORT ANSWER QUESTIONS

1 | **Describe the maturation and development of the Graafian follicle within the menstrual cycle.**

The hypothalamus: gonadotrophin releasing hormone stimulates the anterior lobe of the pituitary gland to secrete follicle stimulating hormone (FSH) and luteinising hormone (LH).

Follicle stimulating hormone: its target is the ovary. This stimulates the development of primordial follicles into primary follicles; each primary follicle contains an oocyte surrounded by granulosa cells. The zona pellucida separates the oocyte from the granulosa cells. Continued development occurs with differentiation into two layers (theca interna and theca externa) and it is now known as a secondary follicle. The theca interna secretes oestrogens and the granulosa cells secrete follicular fluid. The corona radiata is subsequently formed between the granulosa cells and the zona pellucida. The secondary follicle enlarges eventually turning into a mature graafian follicle.

Luteinising hormone: its target is the ovary. This stimulates the final development of the follicle; it stimulates ovulation, also the development of the corpus luteum which produces progesterone, some oestrogen and relaxin.

2 | **With reference to the menstrual cycle and associated hormones describe the changes which occur in the endometrium.**

There are three phases during the menstrual cycle where the endometrium is affected.

Days 1–5 Menstrual phase – if fertilisation of the ovum has not occurred the corpus luteum degenerates and as a consequence luteinising hormone and progesterone levels decline. The blood vessels of the endometrium go into spasm depriving the endometrial cells of oxygen. As a result the functional layer of the endometrium is shed, with accompanying bleeding.

Days 6–14 Proliferative phase (or follicular phase) – rising oestrogen levels from the ovaries and follicle cause regeneration of the functional layer of the endometrium from the basal layer. There is an increase in glands and vascular supply giving the endometrium a velvety appearance. A surge in luteinising hormone at the end of this phase causes ovulation.

Days 15–28 Secretory phase (or luteal phase) – further increased vascularisation occurs as a result of the corpus luteum of the ovary producing progesterone. Glands in the endometrium increase in size and secrete nutrients in preparation for a potential blastocyst implanting.

This answer is based on a 28 day cycle, though this can vary between 21 and 40 days. The only constant interval in women with different cycles seems to be the time span between ovulation and the menses (the secretory phase).

3 **Describe the preparatory processes the sperm undergoes prior to fertilisation.**

This is known as capacitation. It is a process which takes approximately 7 hours and where the sperm are conditioned while in the female reproductive tract en route to fertilising the ovum. The plasma membrane around the head of the sperm contains cholesterol, glycoproteins and proteins; these are removed. The sperm cannot penetrate the corona radiata or zona pellicida surrounding the ovum until this has happened. The acrosomal membrane disintegrates under the influence of a sperm receptor in the zona pellucida. Consequently two enzymes – acrosyn and hyaluronidase – are released by all the sperm in the area digesting a path through the corona radiata and zona pellucida to the ovum. Usually only one sperm penetrates the zona pellucida and polyspermy is prevented by depolarisation of the cell membrane of the ovum.

4 **Identify the physiological rationale for folic acid recommendation prior to pregnancy.**

Folic acid is synthesised in the gastrointestinal tract by bacteria. It is essential for erythropoiesis and the production of white blood cells. It is also involved in the synthesis of DNA and RNA. Mothers who are deficient in folic acid have an increased risk of having a child with neural tube defect (spina bifida, anencephaly or encephalocele). The neural tube normally develops in the embryonic period (neurulation) from approximately 3 weeks gestation and the primitive brain develops from 4 weeks gestation. Neural tube defects are caused by normal growth and development being interrupted or prevented. Deficiency in folic acid can cause this. In the UK supplementation with folic acid (0.4 mg) has been proved to reduce neural tube defects in the fetus. It should be commenced 3–6 months prior to pregnancy as often the woman will be at least 3–4 weeks into gestation before she suspects pregnancy, by which time neurulation has started to occur. If a woman conceives and has not taken folic acid it should be taken until the 12th week of pregnancy. Also all women should continue to take folic acid until the 12th week of pregnancy as elements of the spinal cord are still developing and growing.

5 An optimal body mass index is recommended prior to pregnancy. How can this be achieved from a balanced diet?

A balanced diet consists of: proteins, carbohydrates, fibre, fats/lipids, water soluble vitamins, fat soluble vitamins, minerals, trace elements and water. Proteins are required for growth and repair of body tissues and are contained in cells, enzymes, hormones, antibodies, muscles and blood. They are classified as fibrous or structural proteins (such as collagen or keratin) and also globular, and play a vital role in biological processes. Within the diet proteins can be identified as complete when they contain all essential amino acids, e.g. any animal protein, and incomplete where the protein contains either small quantities or a limited number of amino acids. Carbohydrates are predominantly plant in origin except for lactose and glycogen. They are classified as monosaccharide, disaccharide and polysaccharide and supply the body with energy for vital organs and are protein sparing. Any excess carbohydrate is initially stored as glycogen.

Lipids are animal and plant in origin. Saturated fats are solid at room temperature and sourced from animals. Unsaturated fats are liquid at room temperature and are further subdivided into mono- and poly-unsaturated fats. The main purposes of fats are protection of some vital organs, insulation, energy and cell membrane competence.

The key to maintaining an optimal BMI of 19–25 is ensuring the volume of ingested food, particularly in relation to carbohydrates and lipids, is equivalent to the individual's energy requirements. Any excess of these will be deposited as fat subcutaneously and within/between the body organs.

6 Describe the process of spermatogenesis.

Spermatogenesis is the formation and development of sperm in the seminiferous tubules in the testes. The process takes 65–70 days. Gonadotrophic releasing hormone from the hypothalamus stimulates the anterior pituitary gland to produce follicle stimulating hormone (FSH) and luteinising hormone (LH) both of which are essential in the process. Spermatogonia at the basement membrane replicate initially by mitosis to keep a constant supply of diploid cells maintained. As they develop and become more mature they move away and towards the lumen of the tubule. Further development by meiosis causes the spermatogonium to differentiate into a primary spermatocyte, then a secondary spermatocyte, then an early spermatid and finally a late spermatid. Each spermatogonium will eventually give rise to four haploid daughter cells (spermatozoa). Amongst the spermatogenic cells are Sertoli cells (sustentacular or nursemaid cells). Amongst other functions these cells nourish, support and protect the developing sperm cells and also mediate the effects of FSH and testosterone. They also produce inhibin which regulates FSH levels and hence spermatogenesis.

LH stimulates the Leydig cells to secrete testosterone, which is synthesised from cholesterol. This can also be converted to a more potent form, dihydrotestosterone (DHT) by target cells in the prostate gland and seminal vesicles. The Leydig cells are between the seminiferous tubules.

FSH indirectly stimulates spermatogenesis and works in combination with testosterone to stimulate the production of androgen binding protein (ABP). ABP binds to the testosterone to keep the level high, close to the exit of the seminiferous tubule where the final stages of sperm maturation (spermiogenesis) occurs prior to ejaculation.

7 **Describe the process of oogenesis.**

Primitive germ cells migrate from the yolk sac to the ovaries and differentiate into oogonia. These oogonia with a diploid number of chromosomes commence the meiotic process in the ova of the fetus from a very early gestation (3–4 weeks). Meiotic arrest occurs during the meiosis I prophase stage. After puberty meiosis I is completed producing a secondary oocyte + first polar body. This secondary oocyte has a haploid number of chromosomes. The secondary oocyte begins meiosis II and again the process is arrested in the metaphase stage. Once this secondary oocyte is released from the ovary, if fertilised meiosis II is completed, the oocyte splits into the ovum and second polar body (which disintegrates).

8 **Describe the implantation of the blastocyst.**

The outer layer of the blastocyst is surrounded by syncitiotrophoblastic cells. These produce a proteolytic enzyme which digests maternal tissue. The blastocyst burrows under the maternal decidua inner cell mass first and usually implants in the anterior or posterior wall of the upper body of the uterus.

9 **Identify the differences between oral progesterone only and oral combined contraception in their action on the menstrual cycle.**

Combined oral contraception (COC) prevents ovulation by suppressing the release of gonadotrophins (FSH and LH). They inhibit follicular development thereby preventing ovulation; this is the primary mechanism of COCs. A secondary action of COCs is to thicken cervical mucus, to prevent penetration of sperm, and to thin the lining of the endometrium and to prevent implantation.

Progesterone only (POP) oral contraception prevents pregnancy by increasing the viscosity of cervical mucus thereby inhibiting penetration of sperm through the cervical canal. It also thins the endometrial lining, inhibiting implantation of a fertilised ovum. This is the primary mechanism of older POPs. A newer type of POP mimics COCs by suppressing ovulation in 97% of cycles in women.

10 **Genetic testing with known parental cystic fibrosis may be offered prior to pregnancy. Describe the inheritance pattern of this autosomal recessive condition for parents who are both carriers of cystic fibrosis.**

The gene for cystic fibrosis is recessive and in genetic convention is written as 'c'. The normal gene is written as 'C'. The genotype for an individual who is a carrier is written as 'Cc' – one normal gene and one affected gene. There is a 50% chance of having a child who is a carrier, a 25% chance of having an unaffected child and a 25% chance of having an affected child.

Mum→	C	c
Dad↓		
C	CC (unaffected)	Cc (carrier)
c	cC (carrier)	Cc (affected)

TRUE OR FALSE?

11 The uterus is anterior to the large bowel. ✔

12 The most fertile time during the menstrual cycle are days 26–28. ✘

The most fertile time is just after ovulation around day 14 prior to the menses.

13 The normal preconception dose for folic acid is 400 mcg daily. ✔

14 The first 14 days of the menstrual cycle is the secretory phase. ✘

The first 14 days of the menstrual cycle is the proliferative phase.

15 Ovulation occurs as a result of a surge in progesterone. ✘

Ovulation occurs as a result of a surge in luteinising hormone.

16 Gonadotrophic releasing hormone (GnRH) is secreted from the hypothalamus. ✔

17 The wall of the uterus consists of three layers, perimetrium, myometrium and endometrium. ✔

18 The perimetrium is shed every month as a result of the menstrual cycle. ✘

The endometrium is shed every month as a result of the menstrual cycle.

19 Sperm are produced in the epididymis. ✘

Sperm are produced in the seminiferous tubules of the testes.

20 Gonadotrophic releasing hormone (GnRH) in the male stimulates the release of follicle stimulating hormone. ✔

MULTIPLE CHOICE
Correct answers identified in bold italics

21 Name one of the ligaments that supports the ovaries, uterus and cervix.

a) cruciate ligament   b) ligamentum teres   c) patellar ligament   *d) round ligament*

22 Which hormone is involved in the menstrual cycle?

a) prolactin   *b) progesterone*   c) pepsin   d) parathyroid hormone

23 Gonadotrophic releasing hormone (GnRH) stimulates the release of which hormone from the following?

a) progesterone   b) oestrogen   *c) luteinising hormone*   d) prolactin

24 Capacitation is a process the sperm undergoes prior to fertilisation. This takes how long?

a) 1 hour   *b) 7 hours*   c) 24 hours   d) 48 hours

25 Which part of the sperm cell is responsible for penetrating the corona radiate of the secondary oocyte for fertilisation to take place?

a) neck   b) flagellum   *c) acrosome*   d) centriole

26 Meiosis is the process of cell division which results in:

a) diploid number of chromosomes   *b) haploid number of chromosomes*
c) replication of identical cells   d) no change to the chromosomes

27 Genotype can be described as:

a) the genetic makeup of an individual   b) the physical features apparent in an individual   c) the blood type of an individual   d) being the same in both parents

28 Which of the following methods of contraception affect the menstrual cycle?

a) condom   b) intrauterine contraceptive device   c) diaphragm   *d) combined oral contraceptive pill*

29 The dimensions of the non pregnant uterus are:

a) 10 cm × 7.5 cm × 5 cm   *b) 7.5 cm × 5 cm × 2.5 cm*   c) 30 cm × 22.5 cm × 20 cm   d) 8 cm × 6 cm × 3 cm

30 **The following is a function of the uterus:**

a) stores urine prior to voiding   b) produces hormones regulating the menstrual cycle   *c) prepares of the endometrium for implantation*   d) forms the placenta

31 **At ovulation the oocyte has developed to what level?**

a) an oogonium   b) a primary oocyte   c) a Graafian follicle
d) a secondary oocyte

32 **Describe the correct position of the uterus:**

a) anteverted and anteflexed   b) retroverted and anteflexed   c) anteverted and retroflexed   d) dextrorotated and anteflexed

33 **Which of the following features is present in the breast prior to pregnancy?**

a) primary areola   b) secondary areola   c) venous engorgement   d) darkening of the areola

34 **On average how many lobes is the breast comprised of?**

a) 18   b) 10   c) 20   *d) 9*

35 **Which of the following is the formula for calculating body mass index?**

a) height divided by weight   *b) weight in grammes divided by height in metres squared*   c) weight divided by height   d) weight squared divided by height

FILL IN THE BLANKS

36 Oestrogen stimulates *growth* of the endometrial lining during the menstrual cycle.

37 Progesterone maintains and further develops the endometrial lining. This is called the *secretory or luteal* phase.

38 Fertilisation generally occurs in the *ampulla* region of the uterine (fallopian) tubule.

39 Ovulation always occurs *14* days prior to the menstrual phase.

40 The variation in days of menstrual cycles between different women is dependent on the length in time of the *proliferative (or follicular)* phase.

41 If fertilisation occurs the effects of progesterone in developing the endometrial lining continues as a result of the blastocyst secreting *human chorionic gonadotrophic* hormone.

42 The genetic material that identifies an individual is called *genotype.*

43 The physical manifestation of genetic material is called *phenotype.*

44 During antenatal screening a *booking* history is taken.

45 Blood supply to the cervix is supplied by the *uterine* and *ovarian* arteries.

LABELLING EXERCISE

Figure 1.1a Uterus

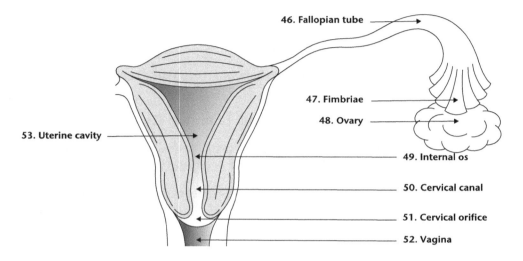

46. Fallopian tube

47. Fimbriae

48. Ovary

53. Uterine cavity

49. Internal os

50. Cervical canal

51. Cervical orifice

52. Vagina

Figure 1.2a Menstrual cycle

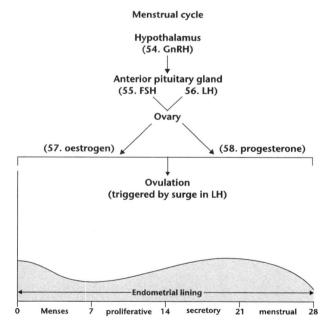

Menstrual cycle

Hypothalamus
(54. GnRH)

Anterior pituitary gland
(55. FSH   56. LH)

Ovary

(57. oestrogen)   (58. progesterone)

Ovulation
(triggered by surge in LH)

Endometrial lining

0   Menses   7   proliferative   14   secretory   21   menstrual   28

Figure 1.3a Sperm

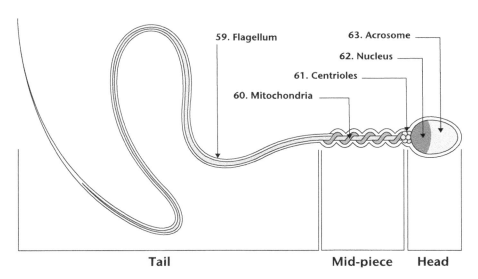

59. Flagellum

63. Acrosome

62. Nucleus

61. Centrioles

60. Mitochondria

Tail   Mid-piece   Head

Figure 1.4a Ovary

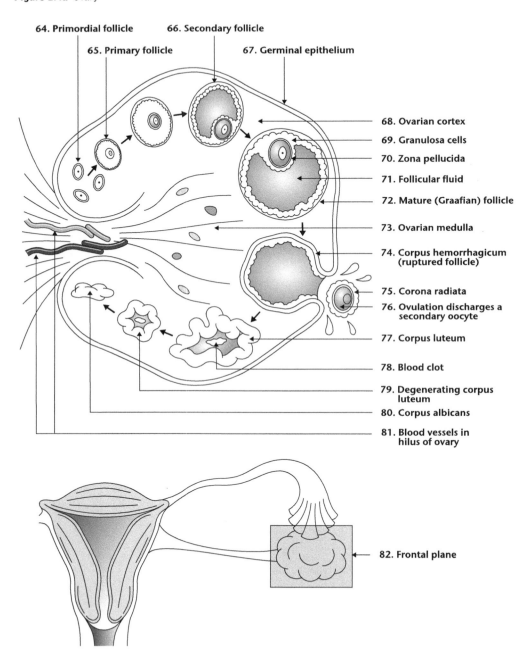

64. Primordial follicle
65. Primary follicle
66. Secondary follicle
67. Germinal epithelium
68. Ovarian cortex
69. Granulosa cells
70. Zona pellucida
71. Follicular fluid
72. Mature (Graafian) follicle
73. Ovarian medulla
74. Corpus hemorrhagicum (ruptured follicle)
75. Corona radiata
76. Ovulation discharges a secondary oocyte
77. Corpus luteum
78. Blood clot
79. Degenerating corpus luteum
80. Corpus albicans
81. Blood vessels in hilus of ovary
82. Frontal plane

Figure 1.5a Genetic inheritance probability pattern

Dad \ Mum	O	O
A	AO	AO
O	OO	OO

2 Pregnancy

SHORT ANSWER QUESTIONS

Write short answers to the following.

1 Describe the non-pregnant cervix. How does it change in pregnancy?

2 State the functions of the placenta.

3 Describe the development of the placenta from the blastocyst to 12 weeks gestation.

4 Describe the changes in the respiratory system during pregnancy.

5 Describe the physiological changes to the uterus which occur as a result of pregnancy.

6 Describe the three components of the midwife's abdominal examination for a woman of 40 weeks gestation. lie, attitude, position.

7 Describe the changes in the renal system in pregnancy.

8 Discuss physiological haemodilution.

9 Describe the changes in the breast during pregnancy.

10 Describe the changes in the skin during pregnancy.

TRUE OR FALSE?

Are the following statements true or false?

11   Erythrocytes increase in number by 50% during pregnancy.

12   Kidney nephrons increase in number during pregnancy.

13   A mild increase in pH of blood occurs in pregnancy.

14   Uterine quiescence during pregnancy occurs due to the effects of oestrogen.

15   Up-regulation and formation of gap junctions in the myometrium occur as a result of increased oestrogen circulation.

16   Oesophageal reflux occurs due to the effects of progesterone on the cardiac sphincter.

17   An increase of hormone levels T3 and T4 are thought to be partly responsible for early nausea/sickness in pregnancy.

18   The breasts produce colostrum from 18 weeks gestation during pregnancy.

19   Kinking of the ureters due to progesterone occurs at the level below the pelvic brim.

20   There is a slight lowering of blood pressure in the second trimester.

a b c d MULTIPLE CHOICE

Identify one correct answer for each of the following.

21 Which of the following is true of oxytocin?

a) It is stored in the adrenal gland

b) It is stored in the anterior pituitary gland

c) It is stored in the hypothalamus gland

d) It is stored in the posterior pituitary gland

22 At 36+ weeks gestation, the fundus of the uterus can be palpated at the level of the:

a) umbilicus

b) xyphisternum

c) symphysis pubis

d) pelvic brim

23 During pregnancy insulin resistance occurs from approximately which week of gestation?

a) 20

b) 12

c) 30

d) 36

24 During the midwife's abdominal palpation the relationship of the fetal spine to the verticle axis of the maternal uterus is known as the:

a) position

b) attitude

c) lie

d) presentation

25 The pelvis has four main variants. Which tends to favour an occipito-posterior position?

a) platypelloid

b) android

c) anthropoid

d) gynaecoid

26 Due to axial displacement of the heart in pregnancy an ECG may show which anomaly?

a) inverted T wave

b) inverted P wave

c) QRS variation

d) inverted Q wave

27 During pregnancy what happens to iron absorption in the mother?

a) It remains the same

b) It is intermittent

c) It decreases

d) It increases

28 Dilution of plasma proteins in maternal circulating blood causes which clinical feature?

a) increase in blood pressure

b) physiological oedema

c) increased urine production

d) decreased circulating blood volume

29 Chloasma occurs as a result of an increase of which circulating hormone?

a) adrenocorticotrophic hormone

b) thyroid stimulating hormone

c) melanocyte stimulating hormone

d) follicle stimulating hormone

30 Which of the following occurs within the gastrointestinal system as a result of progesterone and relaxin hormonal effects?

a) syncope

b) chloasma

c) pica

d) constipation

31 Which of the following foods is recommended as safe to eat during pregnancy?

a) alcohol

b) Brie cheese

c) fruit and vegetables

d) tuna fish

32 Which of the following triglicerides is most implicated in cardiovascular disease?

a) low density lipoprotein

b) very low density lipoprotein

c) high density lipoprotein

d) very high density lipoprotein

33 Which of the following foods is classed as a first class/complete protein?

a) lentils

b) milk

c) meat

d) soya

34 Which of the following is a steroidal hormone produced by the placenta?

a) oestrogen

b) human chorionic gonadotrophin

c) Schwangerschaft's protein

d) human placental lactogen

35 During embryonic development the umbilical cord originates from which of the following?

a) bilaminar disc

b) syncitiotrophoblastic cells

c) the amniotic cavity

d) allantois

FILL IN THE BLANKS

Fill in the blanks in each statement using the options in the box.

increased	oblique/living ligatures
carbon dioxide	human chorionic gonadotrophin
30 cm x 22.5 cm x 20 cm	16
reduced	increases
left	right
increased	

36 There are three layers of muscle fibres in the myometrium. The middle layers are also known as _____ _____.

37 The non-pregnant uterus measures 7.5 cm × 5 cm × 2.5 cm. At term these measurements become: ___ cm x ___ cm x ___ cm.

38 Colostrum can be secreted from the mammary glands from ___ week's gestation.

39 Cardiac output is _____ in pregnancy.

40 Arterial blood pressure is _____ in pregnancy.

41 The trophoblast produces _____ _____ _____ in the first 12 weeks of pregnancy, maintaining functions of the corpus luteum.

42   Dextrorotation of the uterus causes the _____ ureter to be more dilated than the _____ in pregnancy.

43   The glomerular filtration rate is _____ in pregnancy.

44   Tidal volume _____ due to expansion of the rib cage in pregnancy.

45   Maternal arterial _____ _____ levels fall in pregnancy resulting in a mild alkalaemia.

LABELLING EXERCISE

Label the following diagrams: the breast, the pregnant uterus, the fetal circulation, the pelvis and the landmarks of the pelvic brim.

46–59   Figure 2.1 Breast

skin	Cooper's ligament
nipple duct	lobules
lobes	subcutaneous fat
intercostal muscle	alveolus (containing acini cells)
retroglandular fat	nipple
lactiferous duct	intraglandular fat
rib	areola

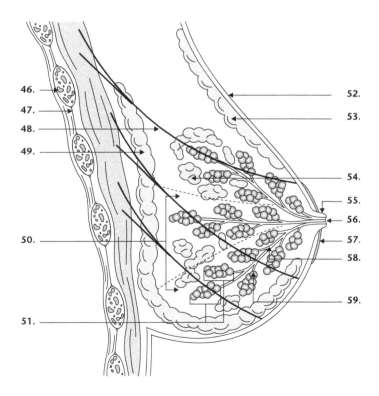

60–62   Figure 2.2 Pregnant uterus

How would the midwife document the findings on abdominal palpation from the diagram below?

> 60. presentation
>
> 61. lie
>
> 62. position

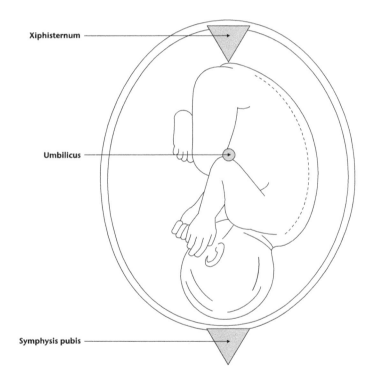

63–73 Figure 2.3 Fetal circulation

descending aorta   superior vena cava

inferior vena cava   umbilical vein

portal vein   ductus arteriosus

umbilical arteries   foramen ovale

internal iliac artery   ductus venosus

hypogastric arteries

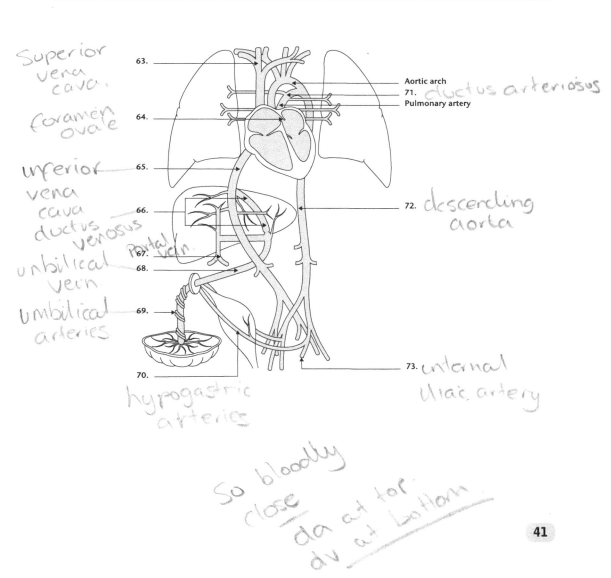

Superior vena cava.

foramen ovale

inferior vena cava ductus venosus

umbilical vein

umbilical arteries

63.

64.

65.

66.

Portal vein.
67.
68.

69.

70.

Aortic arch
71. ductus arteriosus
Pulmonary artery

72. descending aorta

73. internal iliac artery

hypogastric arteries

So bloodly close
da at top
dv at bottom

74–85 Figure 2.4 Pelvis

---

sacrum   sacroiliac joint

iliac crest   coccyx

acetabulum   ischium

ilium   pubic symphysis

pelvic brim   ischial spine

pubic bone

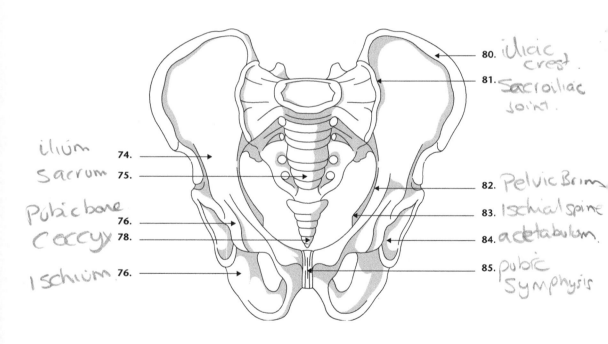

ilium 74.

sacrum 75.

pubic bone 76.

coccyx 78.

ischium 76.

80. iliac crest.

81. Sacroiliac joint.

82. Pelvic Brim

83. Ischial spine

84. acetabulum.

85. pubic symphysis

100%

86–93   Figure 2.5 Landmarks of the pelvic brim

sacral ala (wing)

superior ramus of the pubic bone

sacral promontory

upper inner border of the symphysis pubis

upper inner border of the body of the pubic bone

ileopectineal eminence

ileopectineal line

sacroiliac joint

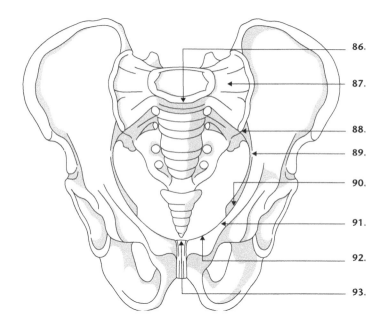

86.

87.

88.

89.

90.

91.

92.

93.

ANSWERS

SHORT ANSWER QUESTIONS

1 **Describe the non pregnant cervix. How does it change in pregnancy?**

There are three layers to the cervix. The lining of endometrium is arranged in folds and looks like a tree, hence the name arbor vitae. It plays no part in menstruation. The middle layer is muscle. The inner circular muscles are thickly arranged and important in dilation in labour. The outer longitudinal muscles extend from the body of the uterus and are involved in effacement. Peritoneum then covers the majority of the cervix. The blood supply is via the uterine arteries and corresponding veins. Lymphatic drainage is via the internal iliac and sacral glands. The nerve supply is from the Lee Frankenhauser plexus. The cardinal, pubocervical and uterosacral ligaments support the cervix.

In pregnancy the cervix becomes more vascular creating a cervix which is softer and blue in colour – Jacquemier's sign. The cervical glands secrete more mucus creating a plug called an operculum. Towards the end of pregnancy the cervix becomes much softer and starts to dilate, which is known as ripening.

2 **State the functions of the placenta.**

The acronym S E R P E N T is useful here as the functions are: storage, endocrine, respiration, protection, excretion, nutrition and transfer of substances.

Storage – the placenta stores glycogen, which it metabolises to provide glucose as the fetus requires it until the fetal liver is sufficiently developed to function. It also stores iron and fat soluble vitamins.

Endocrine – the placenta produces steroid hormones (oestrogen and progesterone) and placental protein hormones (H C G, H P L, Schwangerschaftsprotein 1, P A P P-A, P A P P-B and placental protein 5).

Respiration – oxygen and carbon dioxide is transferred to and from maternal the circulation and to and from the fetus by diffusion. Transfer is assisted by slight maternal respiratory alkalosis in pregnancy. Fetal uptake is assisted by the higher affinity to oxygen of fetal haemoglobin and high fetal haemoglobin levels in utero.

Protection – the placenta acts a filter to most bacteria – however treponema pallidum and tubercle bacilli may transfer to the fetus. Many viruses can transfer, e.g. rubella, parvovirus B19, cytomegalovirus, HIV and hepatitis. Also some protozoa can transfer across the placenta, e.g. malaria, toxoplasmosis.

The placenta filters substances of a high molecular weight, therefore some drugs and medicines may pass through to the fetus. Heparin is filtered. Immunoglobulins will be transferred from mother to fetus in late pregnancy conferring about 6–12 weeks passive immunity to the newborn. In the case of rhesus disease if sensitisation occurs and fetal blood enters the maternal circulation, responding antibodies produced by the mother may cross the placenta and destroy fetal surface antigens and consequently fetal cells.

Excretion – CO_2 is the main product excreted from the fetus. Bilirubin is also excreted due to turnover of red blood cells. Small amounts of urea and uric acid are also excreted.

Nutrition – the fetus receives simplified raw materials for growth and development: protein the in form of amino acids, carbohydrate in the form of glucose, fats in the form of fatty acids and fat soluble vitamins in later stages of pregnancy. Water, vitamins and minerals (e.g. Ca) are also made available to the fetus.

Transfer of substances – the usual cellular membrane transport systems are used: simple diffusion of lipid soluble substances, water pores transfer water soluble substances; facilitated diffusion of glucose using carrier proteins; active transport against concentration gradients of ions (Ca) and endocytosis (pinocytosis) of macromolecules.

3 **Describe the development of the placenta from the blastocyst to 12 weeks gestation.**

The ability of the blastocyst to differentiate into different layers and go on to develop into various aspects of embryo, fetus or placenta is due to the types of cells which exist in the context of human development. Despite now having hundreds of cells the blastocyst is still the same size as the original zygote as it is still encapsulated by the zona pellucida. This is shed prior to implantation. Trophoblasts of the outer cell mass differentiate into three layers: a layer of loose connective tissue known as primitive mesenchyme (this is similar to the mesoderm found in the inner cell mass), and the two are continuous at the point where they join the body stalk. The two other layers of the blastocyst are composed of an inner layer of cytotrophoblasts and an outer layer of syncitiotrophoblasts. Syncitiotrophoblasts produce proteolytic enzymes which digest maternal tissue to help with embedding under the decidua. Cytotrophoblasts secrete HCG which maintains the corpus luteum until the placenta takes over.

The blastocyst implants into the anterior or posterior wall of the body of the uterus and usually with the inner cell mass toward the endometrium. The trophoblasts form into finger-like villi, called chorionic villi and the syncitiotrophoblasts release an enzyme, which breaks down maternal tissue and the spiral endometrial arteries bathing the developing embryo in pools of maternal blood, rich in nutrients. The villi proliferate in the area of the decidua basalis, and this area of the trophoblasts is known as the chorion frondosum which eventually develops into the placenta. These villi also stabilise the placenta and are known as anchoring villi. Other villi, which hang loosely into the maternal blood, are nutritive villi. The villi which are furthest away from the implantation site become smooth and form the chorionic membrane. The amnion is derived from the inner cell mass. The less well-nourished villi which are surrounded by the decidua capsularis degenerate due to lack of nutrition, they become smooth and are known as the chorionic larvae. They eventually become the chorionic membranes.

4   **Describe the changes in the respiratory system during pregnancy.**

Hormonal changes cause capillary engorgement to the mucosa of the respiratory tract. This can cause nasal congestion, voice change and some women may develop an upper respiratory tract infection for the duration of the pregnancy. It can also predispose women to nose bleeds in pregnancy. The diaphragm is upwardly displaced by 4 cm and the anterio-posterior and transverse diameters of the ribcage increase as a result of hormonal effects on the ligaments. This can reduce total lung capacity by 5%. Flaring of ribs occurs (which does not resolve postnatally) and there is a change from abdominal to thoracic breathing.

Oxygen requirements increase by 20% at term; despite this the respiration rate usually remains constant, though may increase by 2–3 respirations per minute. Tidal volume increases and inspirational capacity increases. Expiratory reserve volume (ERV) decreases from the middle of the second trimester. Some women have an increase in vital capacity in pregnancy. Progesterone has a stimulatory effect on the respiratory centre of the medulla oblongata; as a result overbreathing occurs causing alveolar carbon dioxide (CO_2) levels to decrease. Progesterone also causes an increase in carbonic acid anhydrase production in the erythrocytes and this facilitates CO_2 transfer. The result of these changes is a reduced PCO_2 level, potentially leading to a mild respiratory alkalosis, which allows for better gaseous exchange of oxygen (O_2) to the fetus from maternal blood via the placenta and exchange of CO_2 from the fetus to the mother via the placenta and for the CO_2 to be expired from maternal lungs. However this is forestalled by compensatory decreases in sodium bicarbonate from the kidneys.

In the third trimester the enlarging uterus compresses the lower lobes of lungs causing breathlessness.

5   Describe the physiological changes to the uterus which occur as a result of pregnancy.

Increased vascularity to the cervix gives it a bluish colour. The length of 2.5 cm remains constant during pregnancy and the cervix also remains closed. Oestradiol stimulates columnar epithelial growth which can be seen as erosion at the external os and is known as an 'ectropion'. Following conception increased progesterone results in production of mucus forming a plug (operculum) which prevents ascending infection.

The endometrium becomes known as the decidua in pregnancy. Progesterone and oestradiol are mainly responsible for the thickening and increased vascularity in the decidual fundus and upper body of uterus. The decidua alongside trophoblasts also produces relaxin which causes myometrial relaxation.

Oestrogen influences myometrial hyperplasia and hypertrophy; this makes the three layers of the myometrium more clearly defined. Most of the uterine growth is as a result of hypertrophy. The uterus also distends and expands as a result of the growing fetus. The weight of the uterus increases from 50–60 g to 1000 g at term. The sizes increase from 7.5 × 5 × 2.5 cm to 30 × 22.5 × 20 cm at term. Initially the uterine walls are thick but they thin out as pregnancy progresses. There are three muscle layers, the first of which is an outer layer of thin, longitudinal muscle fibres. The middle layer is of spiral (criss-cross) muscle fibres which are interlocked and are slightly thicker and perforated by a network of blood vessels. When these muscle fibres constrict they cause occlusion of the blood vessel and thus prevent haemorrhage to any significant degree following birth. The third layer is the inner circular layers of muscles which form sphincters around the uterine tubules and isthmus. Oestrogens and prostaglandins encourage the formation of gap junctions nearer term which provide electrical connectivity and increase the excitability of the myometrium; this can cause Braxton Hicks contractions to be experienced by the woman. (Overall quiescence is maintained by prostacyclin, progesterone and relaxin.) Nearer to term increased myometrial contractions in the fundus start to draw up the fundal muscle fibres; these pull on the cervix and this causes the beginnings of cervical effacement where the lower segment of the uterus and the cervix become thin and are less contractile.

The perimetrium's folds (the broad ligament) become longer and wider due to the tension caused from the growing uterus. The folds open out to accommodate the enlarged blood vessels and the round ligaments within the perimetrium provide some support for the uterus.

Uterine blood flow increases tenfold, the majority of which perfuses the placenta. A network of arteries develops and penetrates into the decidua and develops into spiral arteries which are remodelled after 16 weeks gestation to become uteroplacental arteries which aid maternal blood flow to the intervillous spaces.

6 | **Describe the three components of the midwife's abdominal examination for a woman of 40 weeks gestation.**

This is comprised of three elements: inspection, palpation and auscultation of the fetal heart.

Inspection – by looking at the abdomen the midwife can assess approximately the size of the uterus. The uterus should change shape from round and globular to long and ovoid as pregnancy progresses, though this may be difficult to visually appreciate in a multiparous woman. The midwife may also notice a saucer-shape depression in the abdomen around the area of the umbilicus indicating the fetus is in an occipito-posterior (OP) position. The umbilicus may protrude as pregnancy advances. Striae gravidarum may be seen, older ones being a silver colour and new ones being red/pink/purple in colour. A brown line known as the linea nigra may also be visible. This line runs from the umbilicus down to the symphysis pubis. Scars will indicate previous obstetric or abdominal surgery and the history of these should be investigated. Care should be taken not to confuse old scarring with elastic marks made from clothing (particularly previous caesarean section scars).

Palpation – the woman should be lying in a semi-recumbent position with hands and arms relaxed by her side. Her abdomen should be exposed to reveal an area from the xiphisternum to the pubic area, while maintaining dignity. Women in advanced pregnancy are subject to supine hypotension due to compression of the inferior vena cava by the fetus and growing uterus. Care should be taken to ensure that if women feel faint they are turned into a left lateral position. Palpation should be systematic commencing with fundal height and proceeding to fundal, lateral and pelvic palpation. To assess the height of the fundus (upper border of the uterus) the midwife should place her hand at the xiphisternum and move it downwards over the abdomen until the curved border of the fundus is found.

To measure the symphysis fundal distance the midwife should place a tape measure at the highest point of the fundus and measure downwards to the upper border of the symphysis pubis (not the pubic hairline). The tape measure should be turned so that the inches side is visible to prevent subjectivity and making the tape measure fit the known weeks of gestation. Once the distance has been measured the tape measure should then be turned over to reveal the measurement in centimetres. The uterus should measure 1 cm per week of gestation between 24 and 37 weeks gestation. A uterus measuring 2 cm less than confirmed weeks of gestation is said to be small for gestational age. A uterus measuring more than 2 cm for the confirmed weeks of gestation is said to be large for gestational age. In both cases further assessment via USS may be necessary. Growth should be plotted on a symphysis-fundal height chart in maternity notes. Other factors which may affect the fundal height are: multiple pregnancy, excess amniotic fluid (polyhydramnios), large or small for gestational age fetus.

Fundal palpation – following assessment of the fundal height, fundal palpation using both hands will determine which part of the fetus (the head or breech) is occupying the upper pole of the uterus. This will also help determine the lie and presentation of the fetus. Buttocks may feel quite broad and firm but they do not feel as hard and round as the fetal head. The fetal head can also be moved independently of the body (balloted), buttocks cannot.

Lateral palpation – the midwife can find the fetal back and as a consequence determine the position of the fetus. Both hands are placed at the sides of the uterus at the level of the umbilicus. By splinting one side of the uterus the midwife can use her other hand to determine whether the continuous resistant line of the fetal spine or the limbs can be felt. The same procedure should be undertaken on the other side. The fetal back can also be located by walking the fingertips over the abdomen from one side to the other.

Pelvic palpation – is used to determine the presentation of the fetus, that is the part of the fetus occupying the lower pole of the uterus. This can be painful for the woman if not undertaken gently. The woman should be asked to bend her knees as this will relax the abdominal muscles. Relaxation may be further aided by undertaking the palpation as the woman slowly breaths out. The fingers of both hands are directed downwards and inwards to determine the fetal part. As with fundal palpation the head will be felt as a round, hard mass (like a cricket ball) compared with a softer broad mass of the buttocks. If the head is in the lower pole (cephalic presentation) the midwife can also assess how much of the fetal head is palpable above the pelvic brim. This is measured in fifths. The head is said to be engaged when 2–3-fifths are palpable above the brim, the remaining 2–3-fifths of the fetal head having descended into the pelvis.

Auscultation of the fetal heart – may confirm that the fetus is alive at that moment in time, but it is of limited value with regards to predictive outcome. The back will have been located during lateral palpation; the midwife will position the pinard stethoscope over the anterior shoulder of the fetus. By placing the pinard at right angles to the abdomen and pressing it gently but firmly against the abdomen, the fetal heart can be heard. It is important to take the woman's pulse at the same time as listening to the fetal heart rate to distinguish between the two and clarify that it is the fetal heart that is being heard and not maternal pulse. The midwife should count the heart rate for a full minute. The heart rate should range between 110 and 160 beats per minute (*Antenatal Care*, NICE 2008).

7   Describe the changes in the renal system in pregnancy.

The kidneys enlarge by 1.5 cm due to an increase of blood flow through them of 35–60%. The blood supply to the kidneys also increases. Frequency of micturition in early pregnancy is related to hormonal changes and increased circulating volume. In late pregnancy it is due to pressure from the engaged presenting part pressing on the bladder. The effects of progesterone cause atonic ureters, which kink and dilate causing urinary stasis, leading to predisposition to urinary tract infections (UTIs). There is an increase in kidney nephron size but not in the actual number. There is an increase in glomerular filtration rate (GFR) by 40–60%, which peaks at about 6–16 weeks gestation. Therefore there is an increase in protein, sugar, folic acid and iodine in urine. Glycosuria occurs as the renal threshold for glucose is reduced and tubular reabsorption cannot keep up with the increased glomerular filtration rate. Dilation of the renal calyces and pelves occurs and also of the ureters in the first trimester; this is more prominent after 20 weeks. The lumen of the ureters increases and hypertrophy of smooth muscle occurs (due to oestrogen) and there is an increase in muscle tone. The ureters elongate and become tortuous and displaced laterally by the growing uterus. The ureters hold 25 times more urine (up to 300 ml). Therefore there is an increased risk of UTI. The ureters below the pelvic brim remain unchanged. The right ureter is usually more dilated than the left due to dextrorotation.

8   Discuss physiological haemodilution.

Maternal blood volume increases in pregnancy by 30–45% to compensate for maternal changes, supplying the uteroplacental–fetal unit and allowing for blood loss in labour. Plasma volume increases by 50% but a relatively smaller increase in red blood cells of 18–25% occurs. The latter is under the influence of erythropoietin. This results in a dilution of red cell concentration creating apparent physiological anaemia. The drop is usually approximately 2g/dl over the pregnancy and is at its lowest at 32 weeks gestation. Serum ferritin levels tend to give a more accurate picture of iron levels than haemoglobin estimation in the first two trimesters of pregnancy. Physiological haemodilution leading to physiological anaemia does not routinely need treating with iron supplementation unless haemoglobin level falls below 10.5g/dl.

9 **Describe the changes in the breast during pregnancy.**

At 4 weeks gestation many women experience tingling and tenderness of the breast as one of the early signs of pregnancy. At 12 weeks there is an increase in size of the breasts and the veins may be more prominent. At 13 weeks skin changes will be noted with the nipple and areola area darkening and the formation of a secondary areola. Montgomery tubercles will also become noticeable on the surface of the areola. Many women will start secreting colostrum at 16 weeks. In late pregnancy the nipple becomes more prominent.

10 **Describe the changes in the skin during pregnancy.**

Striae gravidarum (stretch marks) can appear on the abdomen, thighs and breasts. New stretch marks tend to be red, their colour diminishing over time to a silver colour. Pigmentation increases due to the melanocyte stimulating effects of progesterone and oestrogen and an increase in melanocyte stimulating hormone from the anterior pituitary gland. The areola, nipples, linea nigra (formerly linea alba) and perineum all become darker. Chloasma/melasma (the mask of pregnancy) can be seen on the face and is caused by deposition of melanin in dermal/epidermal macrophages.

Sebaceous glands and sweat glands become more active; this can cause acne in some women. Conversely an increase in cortisol, a natural steroid (from the adrenal cortex), can cause an improvement in some skin conditions during pregnancy. There is an increase in hair growth in pregnancy but following birth this is reversed and lots of hair appears to fall out. Normal hair growth returns usually by 6–12 months postpartum.

TRUE OR FALSE?

11   **Erythrocytes increase in number by 50% during pregnancy.**   ✖

Erythrocytes increase in number by 18–25% during pregnancy.

12   **Kidney nephrons increase in number during pregnancy.**   ✖

Kidney nephrons increase in size during pregnancy.

13   **A mild increase in pH of blood occurs in pregnancy.**   ✔

14   **Uterine quiescence during pregnancy occurs due to the effects of oestrogen.**   ✖

Uterine quiescence during pregnancy occurs due to the effects of progesterone.

15   **Up-regulation and formation of gap junctions in the myometrium occur as a result of increased oestrogen circulation.**   ✔

16   **Oesophageal reflux occurs due to the effects of progesterone on the cardiac sphincter.**   ✔

17   **An increase of hormone levels T3 and T4 are thought to be partly responsible for early nausea/sickness in pregnancy.**   ✔

18   **The breasts produce colostrum from 18 weeks gestation during pregnancy.**   ✖

The breasts produce colostrum from 16 weeks gestation during pregnancy.

19   **Kinking of the ureters due to progesterone occurs at the level below the pelvic brim.**   ✖

Kinking of the ureters due to progesterone occurs at the level above the pelvic brim.

20   **There is a slight lowering of blood pressure in the second trimester.**   ✔

MULTIPLE CHOICE

Correct answers identified in bold italics

21 **Which of the following is true of oxytocin?**

a) It is stored in the adrenal gland   b) It is stored in the anterior pituitary gland   c) It is stored in the hypothalamus gland   *d) It is stored in the posterior pituitary gland*

22 **At 36+ weeks gestation, the fundus of the uterus can be palpated at the level of the:**

a) umbilicus   *b) xyphisternum*   c) symphysis pubis   d) pelvic brim

23 **During pregnancy insulin resistance occurs from approximately which week of gestation?**

a) 20   b) 12   c) 30   d) 36

24 **During the midwife's abdominal palpation the relationship of the fetal spine to the verticle axis of the maternal uterus is known as the:**

a) position   b) attitude   *c) lie*   d) presentation

25 **The pelvis has four main variants. Which tends to favour an occipito-posterior position?**

a) platypelloid   *b) android*   c) anthropoid   d) gynaecoid

26 **Due to axial displacement of the heart in pregnancy an ECG may show which anomaly?**

a) inverted T wave   b) inverted P wave   c) QRS variation   d) inverted Q wave

27 **During pregnancy what happens to iron absorption in the mother?**

a) It remains the same   b) It is intermittent   c) It decreases   *d) It increases*

28 **Dilution of plasma proteins in maternal circulating blood causes which clinical feature?**

a) increase in blood pressure   *b) physiological oedema*   c) increased urine production   d) decreased circulating blood volume

29 Chloasma occurs as a result of an increase of which circulating hormone?

a) adrenocorticotrophic hormone   b) thyroid stimulating hormone
c) melanocyte stimulating hormone   d) follicle stimulating hormone

30 Which of the following occurs within the gastrointestinal system as a result of progesterone and relaxin hormonal effects?

a) syncope   b) chloasma   c) pica   *d) constipation*

31 Which of the following foods is recommended as safe to eat during pregnancy?

a) alcohol   b) Brie cheese   *c) fruit and vegetables*   d) tuna fish

32 Which of the following triglicerides is most implicated in cardiovascular disease?

a) low density lipoprotein   *b) very low density lipoprotein*   c) high density lipoprotein   d) very high density lipoprotein

33 Which of the following foods is classed as a first class/complete protein?

a) lentils   b) milk   *c) meat*   d) soya

34 Which of the following is a steroidal hormone produced by the placenta?

a) oestrogen   b) human chorionic gonadotrophin   c) Schwangerschaft's protein
d) human placental lactogen

35 During embryonic development the umbilical cord originates from which of the following?

a) bilaminar disc   b) syncitiotrophoblastic cells   c) the amniotic cavity
d) allantois

FILL IN THE BLANKS

36 There are three layers of muscle fibres in the myometrium. The middle layers are also known as *oblique/living ligatures.*

37 The non-pregnant uterus measures 7.5 cm × 5 cm × 2.5 cm. At term these measurements become: *30 cm × 22.5 cm × 20 cm.*

38 Colostrum can be secreted from the mammary glands from *16* weeks gestation.

39 Cardiac output is *increased* in pregnancy.

40 Arterial blood pressure is *reduced* in pregnancy.

41 The trophoblast produces *human chorionic gonadotrophin* in the first 12 weeks of pregnancy, maintaining functions of the corpus luteum.

42 Dextrorotation of the uterus causes the *right* ureter to be more dilated than the *left* in pregnancy.

43 The glomerular filtration rate is *increased* in pregnancy.

44 Tidal volume *increases* due to expansion of the rib cage in pregnancy.

45 Maternal arterial *carbon dioxide* levels fall in pregnancy resulting in a mild alkalaemia.

LABELLING EXERCISE

Figure 2.1a Breast

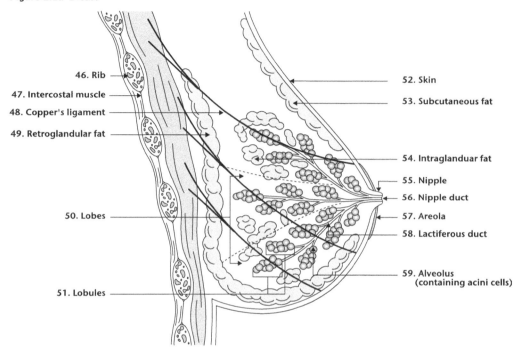

46. Rib
47. Intercostal muscle
48. Copper's ligament
49. Retroglandular fat

50. Lobes

51. Lobules

52. Skin
53. Subcutaneous fat

54. Intraglanduar fat
55. Nipple
56. Nipple duct
57. Areola
58. Lactiferous duct

59. Alveolus
(containing acini cells)

Figure 2.2a Pregnant uterus

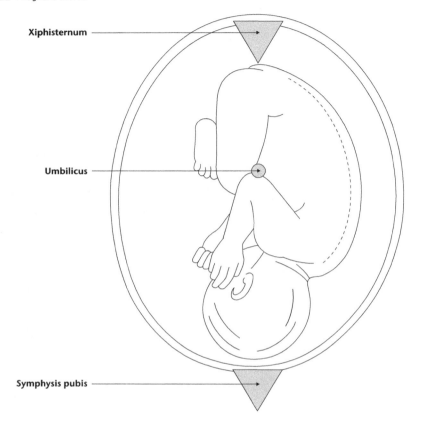

Xiphisternum

Umbilicus

Symphysis pubis

60. presentation = cephalic

61. lie = longitudinal

62. position = left occipito-anterior

Figure 2.3a Fetal circulation

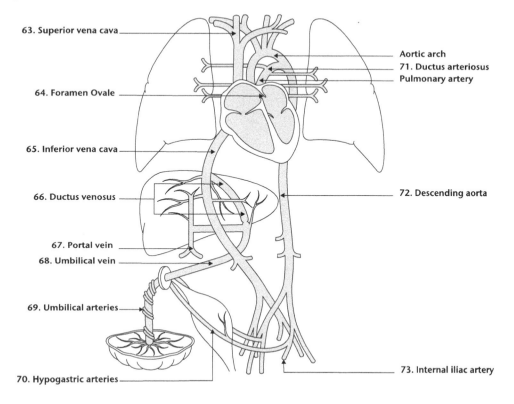

63. Superior vena cava

Aortic arch
71. Ductus arteriosus
Pulmonary artery

64. Foramen Ovale

65. Inferior vena cava

66. Ductus venosus

72. Descending aorta

67. Portal vein
68. Umbilical vein

69. Umbilical arteries

73. Internal iliac artery

70. Hypogastric arteries

Figure 2.4a Pelvis

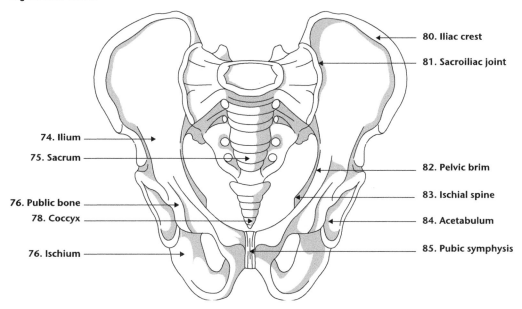

80. Iliac crest
81. Sacroiliac joint
74. Ilium
75. Sacrum
82. Pelvic brim
83. Ischial spine
76. Public bone
78. Coccyx
84. Acetabulum
76. Ischium
85. Pubic symphysis

Figure 2.5a Landmarks of the pelvic brim

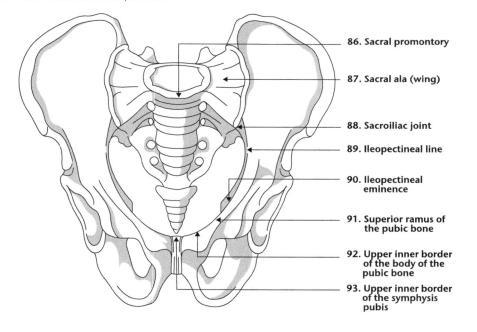

86. Sacral promontory
87. Sacral ala (wing)
88. Sacroiliac joint
89. Ileopectineal line
90. Ileopectineal eminence
91. Superior ramus of the pubic bone
92. Upper inner border of the body of the pubic bone
93. Upper inner border of the symphysis pubis

3 Labour

SHORT ANSWER QUESTIONS

Write short answers to the following.

1 Define the first stage of labour. Describe the physiological processes expected in the uterus during this stage.

2 With regard to vaginal examination describe the changes which may be found during the first and second stages of labour.

3 Describe the differences in diameters and appearance between the four pelvic variants.

4 Describe the differences between caput succedaneum and cephalhaematoma.

5 State the intracranial membranes and sinuses within the fetal skull. Discuss the importance of these structures in midwifery practice.

6 Define the second stage of labour. Discuss the mechanism of the second stage of labour.

7 The perineal body is comprised of which muscles?

8 Describe the mechanism of placental separation.

9 Define the third stage of labour. How may the midwife assess normality of the third stage of labour?

10 What anatomical variations may the midwife find during examination of the placenta and membranes following birth?

TRUE OR FALSE?

Are the following statements true or false?

11 Fundal dominance emanates from the lower uterine segment.

12 Synchronicity is the coordinated action of the myometrium.

13 Engagement of the presenting part is identified as 4/5 palpable.

14 On vaginal examination zero station +3 cm refers to the presenting part being 3 cm above the ischial spines.

15 ROP is abbreviated from right occipito-posterior position.

16 The pubococcygeus muscle is one of the superficial muscles of the pelvic floor.

17 A third degree tear only involves trauma to the skin.

18 Syntometrine only acts on the fundal area of the uterus.

19 Velamentous insertion of the cord passes through the placental membranes.

20 The periosteum is the lowermost part of the fetal skull.

a b c d   MULTIPLE CHOICE

Identify one correct answer for each of the following.

21 During labour uterine contractions are initiated from:

a) the cervix

b) the fetus

c) the cornua

d) the isthmus

22 The normal range of the fetal heart is:

a) 110–150 bpm

b) 110–160 bpm

c) 90–130 bpm

d) 140–170 bpm

23 The gate theory of pain relief is utilised in the use of:

a) epidural

b) pethidine

c) transcutaneous electrical nerve stimulation

d) hypnosis

24 The latent phase of the first stage of labour is described when:

a) contractions are 4 in every 10 minutes

b) cervical dilatation is 3–4 cm

c) cervical dilatation is 9 cm

d) it lasts for 2 hours maximum

25 During the second stage of labour, the occiput on reaching the pelvic floor rotates anteriorly by:

a) 1/8

b) 2/8

c) 3/8

d) 0/8

26 In a well-flexed head the presenting diameter is:

a) mentovertical

b) sub-occipito bregmatic

c) sub-occipito frontal

d) frontal

27 The occipitofrontal diameter is:

a) 11.5 cm

b) 11 cm

c) 9.5 cm

d) 13 cm

28 Blood loss in the third stage of labour is physiologically controlled by:

a) full bladder

b) low levels of oxytocin

c) living ligatures

d) haemodilution

29 An episiotomy involves the following structures:

a) cervix

b) external anal meatus

c) iliococcygeus

d) transverse perinei

30 During the midwife's examination of the placenta the amnion:

a) is friable

b) pulls back to the lateral edge of the placenta

c) is dull

d) is continuous with the umbilical cord

31 What is the role of prostaglandin in labour?

a) acts on the myometrium causing contractions

b) hardens the cervix

c) acts on the perimetrium causing contractions

d) acts on the perineum

32 Which of the following hormones is involved in Ferguson's reflex?

a) oestrogen

b) progesterone

c) prolactin

d) oxytocin

33 What is the physiological importance of the resting tone between contractions?

a) defines incoordinate uterine activity

b) gives the mother a rest

c) allows perfusion of the placenta

d) reduces oxygen levels to the fetus

34 How are the forewaters formed?

a) The amnion separates from the decidua

b) The chorion separates from the decidua

c) The fetus traps liquor behind it

d) As a result of the cervix effacing

35 What structure is involved in a tentorial tear?

a) superior longitudinal sinus

b) inferior longitudinal sinus

c) tentorium cerebellum

d) great vein of Galen

FILL IN THE BLANKS

Fill in the blanks in each statement using the options in the box.

dilatation	upwardly
Lee Frankenhauser	15
fetal	platelets
axis pressure	fetal position
length	contract
Valsalva	spines
consistency	anteriorly
retract	effacement

36 Fetal _____ _____ is the force of fundal pressure which is transferred to the upper pole of the fetus.

37 Longitudinal muscle fibres of the myometrium _____ and _____ during labour.

38 Zero station is the landmark of the ischial _____ from which fetal descent can be assessed.

39 Cervical assessment includes the five components of the modified Bishop's score which includes: _____, _____, _____, _____ and _____.

40 Intermittent auscultation of the fetal heart in the active phase of the first stage of labour occurs every _____ minutes.

41 During labour the bladder is displaced _____ and _____ out of the pelvis.

42   Directed pushing involves the _____ technique which reduces oxygen supply to mother and fetus.

43   The _____ _____ plexus is stimulated during spontaneous pushing in the second stage of labour.

44   _____ increase at the time of birth to help with haemostasis.

45   The Schultz method of placental separation leads to the _____ surface being delivered first.

LABELLING EXERCISE

Label the following diagrams: reflex arc and nerve supply to the uterus, macrostructure of the uterus, muscle layers of the myometrium, superficial and deep muscles of the perineum, the fetal skull and descent of the fetal head in relation to the pelvic brim.

46–49   Figure 3.1 Pain pathway – reflex arc and nerve supply to uterus

anterior aspect of spinal cord   sensory nerve ending in skin receptor

posterior root ganglion   posterior (dorsal) horn

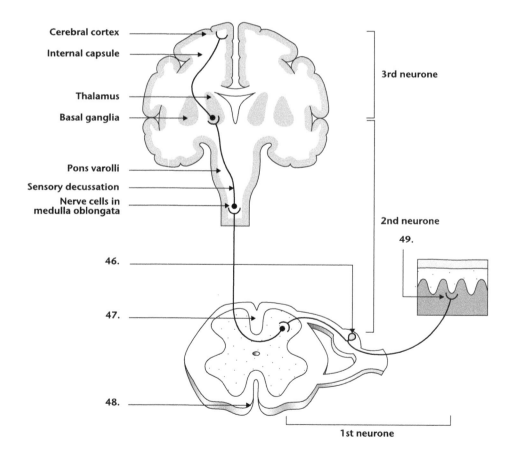

50–56   Figure 3.2 Uterus

cavity	fundus
isthmus	infra-vaginal cervix
cornua	Corpus
supra-vaginal cervix	

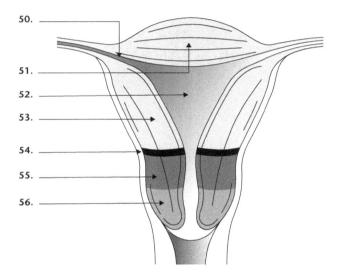

50.
51.
52.
53.
54.
55.
56.

57–59   Figure 3.3 Uterus: identify the muscle structure of the myometrium

middle layer of interlacing oblique fibres

inner layer of circular fibres

outer layer of longitudinal fibres

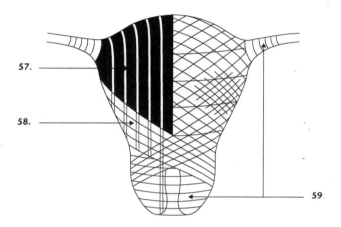

57.

58.

59.

60–81   Figure 3.4 Perineal floor × 2 layers (superficial and deep)

ischiocavernosus	coccyx
urethral orifice	pubococcygeus
rectum	ischial tuberosity
ischial spine	membranous sphincter of the urethra
symphysis pubis	symphysis pubis
coccyx	triangular ligament
clitoris	bulbocavernosus
iliococcygeus	urethra
external anal sphincter	vagina
anus	transverse perineal muscle
vaginal orifice	ischiococcygeus

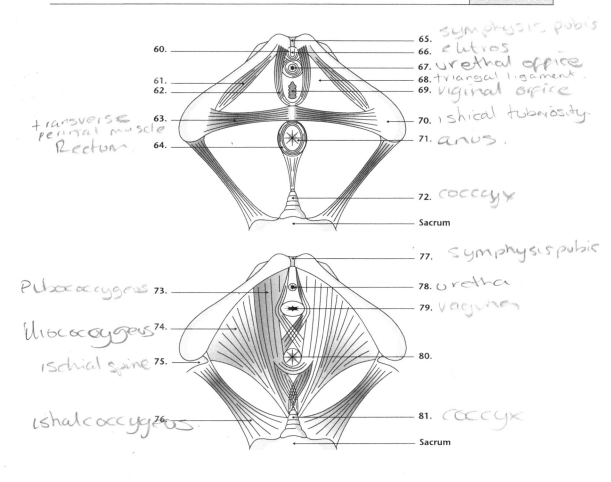

60. _____
61. _____
62. _____
63. _____
64. _____

65. symphysis pubis
66. clitros
67. urethal office
68. triangal ligament.
69. viginal orfice
70. ishical tuberosity.
71. anus.
72. coccyx
Sacrum

transverse perinal muscle
Rectum

Pubococcygeus 73. _____
Uiocacoygeus 74. _____
ischial spine 75. _____
ishalcoccygeus 76. _____

77. symphysis pubis
78. uretha
79. vagina
80. _____
81. coccyx
Sacrum

82–96   Figure 3.5 Fetal skull

parietal bone	occipital bone
frontal bone	anterior fontanelle
lambdoidal suture	sagittal suture
anterior fontanelle	frontal bone
temporal bone	parietal bone
occipital bone	coronal suture
posterior fontanelle	posterior fontanelle
frontal suture	

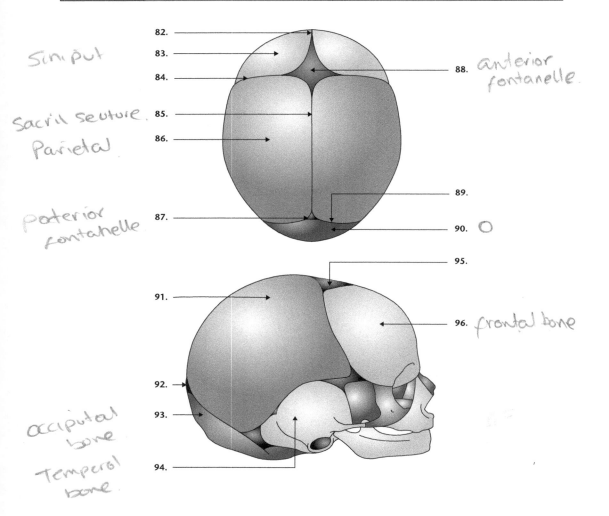

Siniput

Sacril seuture.
Parietal

poterior
fontahelle

occiputal
bone

Temperol
bone.

82.
83.
84.
85.
86.
87.

88. anterior
fontanelle.

89.
90. ○

91.
92.
93.
94.

95.
96. frontal bone

97–108 Figure 3.6 Pelvis – descent of the head

Identify the fifths palpable for each picture and insert an anatomical description.

4/5	Sinciput prominent Occiput descending
Sinciput not so prominent	2/5
head on pelvic floor	Sinciput Occiput not felt
5/5	Sinciput rising Occiput can be tipped
1/5	3/5
Sinciput and Occiput above the brim	0/5

97.	98.	99.	100.	101.	102.
103.	104.	105.	106.	107.	108.

Brim

0/5   1/5   2/5   3/5   4/5   5/5

Sinciput and occiput above the brim

Sinciput occiput not felt.

ANSWERS

SHORT ANSWER QUESTIONS

1 **Define the first stage of labour. Describe the physiological processes expected in the uterus during this stage.**

The first stage of labour is from the onset of regular, painful contractions to full dilatation of the os uteri.

The physiological processes are:

- Fundal dominance – contractions start at one of the cornua of the fundus and spread across and downwards. Contractions usually last longer and are more intense in the fundus.

- Contraction and retraction – muscles fibres retain some of the shortening of contraction (retraction). This allows the fetus to be expelled because the upper segment becomes shorter and thicker and the cavity reduces. Outer longitudinal fibres are particularly important as are the inner circular fibres during this stage of labour. The amplitude and duration of contractions increase as labour progresses.

- Polarity – this is the harmony between the two poles of the uterus. The upper pole (upper uterine segment) contracts and retracts to expel the fetus, the lower pole (lower uterine segment) contracts slightly and dilates to facilitate expulsion.

- Fetal axis pressure – the force of the fundal contraction is transmitted to the upper pole of the fetus, down the long axis of the fetus and applied to the presenting part against the cervix. This causes an attitude of flexion of the descending fetal head.

- Ferguson's reflex – contractions cause pressure of the presenting part on the cervix and upper portion of the vagina causing a neuro-hormonal response and a surge of oxytocin, resulting in increased contractions, this is one of nature's few positive feedback loops.

The formation of fore- and hindwaters – as some of the chorion peels away from the decidua close to the dilating cervix, some of the amniotic fluid becomes trapped in front of the fetal head between the skull and the cevix. This is the forewaters; the remaining fluid trapped behind becomes the hindwaters.

General fluid pressure – while the membranes are intact pressure from the contractions is also exerted on the amniotic fluid. Because fluid is not compressible the pressure is equalised throughout the whole uterus and over the fetal body.

Effacement and dilatation of the cervix – contractions cause the cervix to thin then dilate in primigravid women; in multiparous women effacement and dilatation usually occur simultaneously.

2 **With regard to vaginal examination describe the changes which may be found during the first and second stages of labour.**

There is an appearance of a 'show' (operculum) – as labour progresses more show is generally noted. Spontaneous rupture of membranes (SRM) may be evident due to no forewaters being felt (note colour of any liquor if present).

Effacement and dilatation should increase over time. Once the active phase has commenced (4 cm onward) dilatation should be 0.5 cm/hour in primigravid women and 1 cm/hour in multigravid women. By the end of the first stage cervix should be fully effaced and fully dilated (10 cm).

Increased flexion of fetal skull – with a fully flexed head the posterior fontanelle should be palpated. The presenting diameter will be the sub-occipito bregmatic diameter (9.5 cm).

Change of position of the denominator (occiput) in relation to the pelvis can also be felt. Initially the saggital suture of the fetal skull is in transverse diameter (occipito-transverse, OT) but with descent and rotation of the vertex caused by the pelvic floor, the vertex will rotate to occipito-anterior (OA) position where the occiput and posterior fontanelle can be palpated in the left or right anterior part of the pelvis.

There is a change in level of the fetal skull in relation to the ischial spines (zero station). The distance of the vertex in relation to the ischial spines can be assessed in centimetres above spines or below the level of spines. Spines cannot usually be physically palpated on vaginal examination but an estimation is made of where they are. As descent occurs the level of the fetal skull lowers though the birth canal.

Caput and moulding may be noted – the extent of this will determine if labour is progressing normally. Caput and moulding can be more severe due to delay in progress.

3 Describe the differences in diameters and appearance between the four pelvic variants.

Gynaecoid pelvis	Android pelvis
Brim – rounded	Brim – heartshaped
Fore pelvis – generous	Fore pelvis – narrow
Side walls – straight	Fore pelvis – convergent
Ischial spines – blunt	Ischial spines – prominent
Sciatic notch – rounded	Sciatic notch – narrow
Sub-pubic arch – 90°	Sub-pubic arch <90°
Incidence – 50%	Incidence – 20%
Anthropoid	Platypelloid
Brim – long oval	Brim – kidney shaped
Fore pelvis – narrowed	Fore pelvis – wide
Side walls – divergent	Fore pelvis – divergent
Ischial spines – blunt	Ischial spines – blunt
Sciatic notch – wide	Sciatic notch – wide
Sub-pubic arch > 90°	Sub-pubic arch >90°
Incidence – 25% (50% non-Caucasian)	Incidence – 5%

4 Describe the differences between caput succedaneum and cephalhaematoma.

Caput succedaneum occurs with a cephalic presentation and is an oedematous swelling consisting of blood and serous fluid just below the scalp but above the periosteum. Single caput succedaneum can be present and a false one generated by a ventouse birth. This is usually present at birth, does not usually enlarge, will pit on pressure, crosses suture lines and will resolve within 36 hours of birth. The baby may be uncomfortable but careful handling is usually sufficient.

Cephalhaematoma in contrast occurs under the periosteum which covers the skull bones and is indicative of cephalopelvic disproportion, precipitate labour or ventouse birth. Separation of the periosteum from the bone causes bleeding but is limited to one bone. Bilateral cephalhaematomas are therefore possible.

They are not present at birth, appearing around 12 hours after birth and increase in size over the next few days. They can last several weeks. They do not pit with pressure, are fixed and do not cross suture lines. The baby will be uncomfortable and may develop jaundice as the haematoma is broken down.

5 | **State the intracranial membranes and sinuses within the fetal skull. Discuss the importance of these structures in midwifery practice.**

There are two important membranes, the falx cerebri and the tentorium cerebelli. The sinuses or large veins are: the superior saggital sinus, inferior saggital sinus, the great cerebral vein of Galen, two lateral sinuses and the straight sinus.

During labour moulding occurs where the bones of the fetal skull override each other. If the head is subject to abnormal moulding during labour (due to malposition) or if a precipitate labour occurs the sinuses may be put at risk from tearing. The most vulnerable area is the junction between the falx cerebri and the tentorium cerebelli. If this area is torn the great vein of Galen can rupture and cause haemorrhage.

6 | **Define the second stage of labour. Discuss the mechanism of the second stage of labour.**

The second stage of labour extends from the full dilatation of the cervix to the complete birth of the baby. The mechanism of the second stage occurs as the baby negotiates its way through the birth canal using the widest diameters. The following processes occur: descent, flexion, internal rotation, extension of the head, restitution, internal rotation of the shoulders and lateral flexion. Commonly, abdominal palpation will identify a longitudinal lie, cephalic presentation, right or left occipito-anterior position, well-flexed attitude, with the denominator being the occiput.

Descent of the fetus occurs as a consequence of contraction and retraction of the uterine muscles. Fetal axis pressure increases flexion on the head resulting in the suboccipito-bregamatic diameter presenting (9.5 cm) and the occiput leading. As the occiput is pushed onto the pelvic floor, a muscular diaphragm, its resistance creates rotation, usually one-eighth anteriorly. This allows the widest diameter of the pelvis, the anteroposterior to be utilised but creates a twist in the baby's neck. The occiput then slips beneath the sub-pubic arch and crowning occurs when the head no longer recedes between contractions. Following crowning the sinciput, face and chin sweep the perineum and extension occurs as the head is born. Restitution is the realignment of the head and neck. The anterior shoulder then internally rotates on the levator ani muscle in the same direction that restitution had occurred to lie under the symphysis pubis. External rotation of the head is simultaneously seen. In a supported sitting position the anterior shoulder is usually born first followed by the posterior shoulder and lateral flexion sideways following the curve of carus.

7 **The perineal body is comprised of which muscles?**

The perineal body is a pyramid shaped mass of muscular and fibrous tissue between the vagina and rectum, measuring approximately 4 cm along each side. It has an apex and a base, the apex is the deepest part and is formed by the pubococcygeus muscle. The transverse perineal muscles, the bulbocavernosus and the external anal sphincter make up the base.

8 **Describe the mechanism of placental separation.**

Membranes have started to separate in the first stage of labour when the chorion detaches slightly and causes some bleeding which makes up part of the show; their separation is completed as the weight of the descending placenta causes them to completely separate.

The process begins with the contraction which delivers the baby's trunk. Separation occurs in the spongy, decidual layer. The placenta is compressed and blood in the intervillous spaces is forced back into the decidual layer. It is prevented from returning to the maternal system by the oblique muscles compressing the uterine blood vessels. These vessels become congested and burst with the next contraction; this causes bleeding between the decidual layer and the maternal surface of the placenta, stripping it away from its attachment.

There are two two methods of separation: Schultz and Matthews Duncan.

Schultz is most common; this starts in centre of the placenta, a retroplacental clot is formed, the fetal surface appears at the vulva and the membranes trail behind. This method is associated with less bleeding. In the Matthews Duncan method no retroplacental clot is formed and separation starts from the lower edge. The placenta slips down and maternal surface is seen at the vulva. The separation is usually slower and more bleeding is usually evident.

9 **Define the third stage of labour. How may the midwife assess normality of the third stage of labour?**

The third stage of labour extends from the birth of the baby to the full expulsion of the placenta and membranes and confirmation of haemostasis. This can last from 5–15 minutes particularly in active management of the third stage or up to an hour physiologically.

Following the birth of the baby, the uterus continues to contract reducing the surface and forcing the inelastic placenta to shear off the uterine wall. Abdominally the uterus then rises as the placenta falls into the lower segment. A trickle of blood or extension of the cord may also be noted. Separation usually occurs centrally following the formation of a retroplacental clot with the fetal surface then presenting first – this process is called the Schultz method of separation. Haemostasis is achieved by oblique uterine muscle fibres acting as clamps of the bleeding vessels, strong contraction of the uterus causing apposition of the walls and a temporary activation of the coagulation and fibrinolitic systems support clot formation.

Examination of the placenta and membranes for completeness, the vagina and perineum for trauma and estimation of blood loss are essential to the assessment of normality in the third stage.

10   **What anatomical variations may the midwife find during examination of the placenta and membranes following birth?**

A succenturiate lobe is an extra lobe or lobes connected to the placenta by a blood vessel running through the membranes. It is important to check around the edges of the placenta and membranes to ensure there are no vessels leading off the main placenta. If a lobe is missing from this vessel it probably has been retained in utero, this could lead to infection and/or haemorrhage.

A bipartite or tripartite placenta – here the placenta is divided into two or three separate placentae. Each have their own cord which join part way up the main umbilical cord – this is of no clinical significance.

A circumvallate placenta is where an opaque thick moat-like ring running around the edge of placenta. It is seen on the fetal surface where the membranes have doubled back on themselves. This has been associated with an increased risk of IUGR.

Placental infarcts are localised areas of death of placental tissue; new infarcts are red which degenerate into white patches. They are commonly associated with hypertension and smoking. Areas of calcification are gritty white/grey patches and are common in post-mature placentae; they are of no clinical significance.

A velamentous insertion of umbilical cord is where the cord is inserted into membranes rather than placenta directly. This leaves exposed fetal vessels running across and through the membranes. It can cross the internal os causing a vasa praevia. Subsequent rupture of these vessels can cause an extreme fetal haemorrhage.

A battledore placenta occurs when the cord is inserted into the edge of the placenta.

TRUE OR FALSE?

11 **Fundal dominance emanates from the lower uterine segment.**

Fundal dominance emanates from the upper uterine segment.

12 **Synchronicity is the coordinated action of the myometrium.**

13 **Engagement of the presenting part is identified as 4/5 palpable.**

Engagement of the presenting part is when the fetal head is 2/5 palpable.

14 **On vaginal examination zero station +3 cm refers to the presenting part being 3 cm above the ischial spines.**

On vaginal examination zero station +3 cm refers to the presenting part being 3 cm below the ischial spines.

15 **ROP is abbreviated from right occipito-posterior position.**

16 **The pubococcygeus muscle is one of the superficial muscles of the pelvic floor.**

The pubococcygeus muscle is one of the deep muscles of the pelvic floor.

17 **A third degree tear only involves trauma to the skin.**

A third degree tear involves trauma to the skin, the superficial and deep perineal muscles with partial or complete disruption of the anal sphincter muscles (which may involve the external and the internal sphincter muscles).

18 **Syntometrine only acts on the fundal area of the uterus.**

Syntometrine is a general vasoconstrictor so it will have some effect on the lower uterine segment as well as the fundus.

19 **Velamentous insertion of the cord passes through the placental membranes.**

20 **The periosteum is the lowermost part of the fetal skull.**

MULTIPLE CHOICE
Correct answers identified in bold italics

21 **During labour uterine contractions are initiated from:**

a) the cervix   b) the fetus   *c) the cornua*   d) the isthmus

22 **The normal range of the fetal heart is:**

a) 110–150 bpm   *b) 110–160 bpm*   c) 90–130 bpm   d) 140–170 bpm

23 **The gate theory of pain relief is utilised in the use of:**

a) epidural   b)pethidine   *c) transcutaneous electrical nerve stimulation*
d) hypnosis

24 **The latent phase of the first stage of labour is described when:**

a) contractions are 4 in every 10 minutes   *b) cervical dilatation is 3–4 cm*
c) cervical dilation is 9 cm   d) it lasts for 2 hours maximum

25 **During the second stage of labour, the occiput on reaching the pelvic floor rotates anteriorly by:**

a) 1/8   b) 2/8   c) 3/8   d) 0/8

26 **In a well-flexed head the presenting diameter is:**

a) mentovertical   *b) sub-occipito bregmatic*   c) sub-occipito frontal   d) frontal

27 **The occipitofrontal diameter is:**

a) 11.5 cm   b) 11 cm   c) 9.5 cm   d) 13 cm

28 **Blood loss in the third stage of labour is physiologically controlled by:**

a) full bladder   b) low levels of oxytocin   *c) living ligatures*   d) haemodilution

29 **An episiotomy involves the following structures:**

a) cervix   b) external anal meatus   c) iliococcygeus   *d) transverse perinei*

30 **During the midwife's examination of the placenta the amnion:**

a) is friable   b) pulls back to the lateral edge of the placenta   c) is dull
d) is continuous with the umbilical cord

31 **What is the role of prostaglandin in labour?**

a) acts on the myometrium causing contractions   b) hardens the cervix
c) acts on the perimetrium causing contractions   d) acts on the perineum

32 **Which of the following hormones is involved in Ferguson's reflex?**

a) oestrogen   b) progesterone   c) prolactin   *d) oxytocin*

33 **What is the physiological importance of the resting tone between contractions?**

a) defines incoordinate uterine activity   b) gives the mother a rest
c) allows perfusion of the placenta   d) reduces oxygen levels to the fetus

34 **How are the forewaters formed?**

a) The amnion separates from the decidua   *b) The chorion separates from the decidua*   c) The fetus traps liquor behind it   d) As a result of the cervix effacing

35 **What structure is involved in a tentorial tear?**

a) superior longitudinal sinus   b) inferior longitudinal sinus   c) tentorium cerebellum   *d) the great vein of Galen*

FILL IN THE BLANKS

36 Fetal *axis pressure* is the force of fundal pressure which is transferred to the upper pole of the fetus.

37 Longitudinal muscle fibres of the myometrium *contract* and *retract* during labour.

38 Zero station is the landmark of the ischial *spines* from which fetal descent can be assessed.

39 Cervical assessment includes the five components of the modified Bishop's score which includes: *length, fetal position, consistency, effacement* and *dilatation.*

40 Intermittent auscultation of the fetal heart in the active phase of the first stage of labour occurs every *15* minutes.

41 During labour the bladder is displaced *upwardly* and *anteriorly* out of the pelvis.

42 Directed pushing involves the *Valsalva* technique which reduces oxygen supply to mother and fetus.

43 The *Lee Frankenhauser* plexus is stimulated during spontaneous pushing in the second stage of labour.

44 *Platelets* increase at the time of birth to help with haemostasis.

45 The Schultz method of placental separation leads to the *fetal* surface being delivered first.

LABELLING EXERCISE

Figure 3.1a Pain pathway

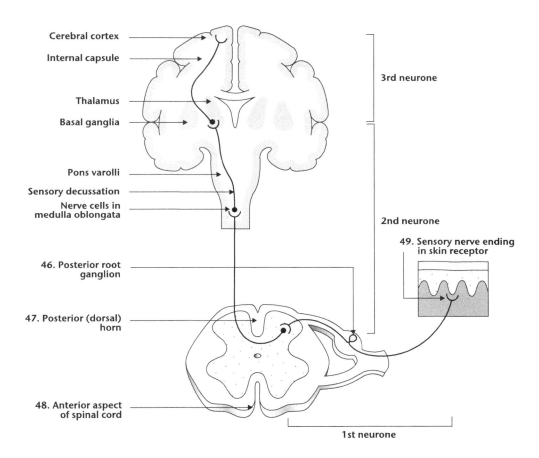

Cerebral cortex

Internal capsule

Thalamus

Basal ganglia

3rd neurone

Pons varolli

Sensory decussation

Nerve cells in
medulla oblongata

2nd neurone

49. Sensory nerve ending
in skin receptor

46. Posterior root
ganglion

47. Posterior (dorsal)
horn

48. Anterior aspect
of spinal cord

1st neurone

Figure 3.2a Uterus

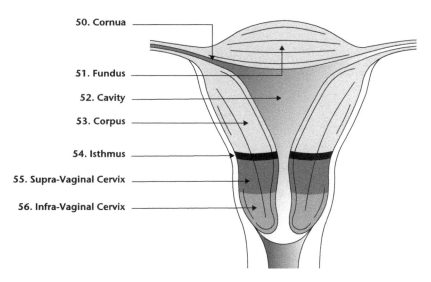

50. Cornua
51. Fundus
52. Cavity
53. Corpus
54. Isthmus
55. Supra-Vaginal Cervix
56. Infra-Vaginal Cervix

Figure 3.3a Uterus

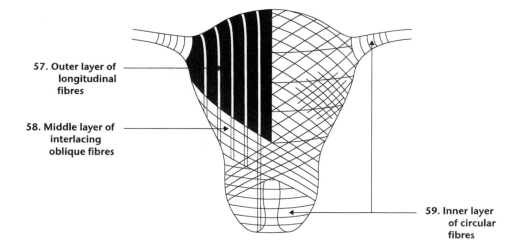

57. Outer layer of longitudinal fibres
58. Middle layer of interlacing oblique fibres
59. Inner layer of circular fibres

Figure 3.4a Perineal floor × 2 layers

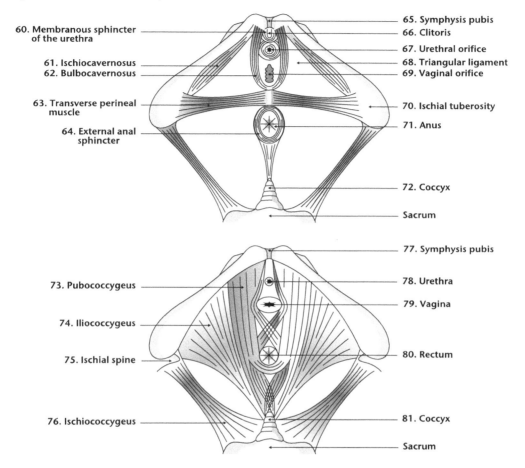

60. Membranous sphincter of the urethra
61. Ischiocavernosus
62. Bulbocavernosus
63. Transverse perineal muscle
64. External anal sphincter

65. Symphysis pubis
66. Clitoris
67. Urethral orifice
68. Triangular ligament
69. Vaginal orifice
70. Ischial tuberosity
71. Anus
72. Coccyx
Sacrum

73. Pubococcygeus
74. Iliococcygeus
75. Ischial spine
76. Ischiococcygeus

77. Symphysis pubis
78. Urethra
79. Vagina
80. Rectum
81. Coccyx
Sacrum

Figure 3.5a Fetal skull

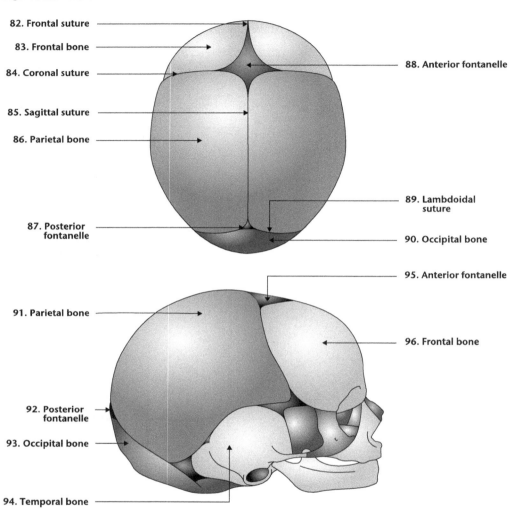

82. Frontal suture
83. Frontal bone
84. Coronal suture
85. Sagittal suture
86. Parietal bone
87. Posterior fontanelle
88. Anterior fontanelle
89. Lambdoidal suture
90. Occipital bone
95. Anterior fontanelle
91. Parietal bone
96. Frontal bone
92. Posterior fontanelle
93. Occipital bone
94. Temporal bone

Figure 3.6a Pelvis – descent of the head

97. $\frac{5}{5}$	98. $\frac{4}{5}$	99. $\frac{3}{5}$	100. $\frac{2}{5}$	101. $\frac{1}{5}$	102. $\frac{0}{5}$
103. Sinciput & Occiput above the brim	104. Sinciput prominent Occiput descending	105. Sinciput rising Occiput can be tipped	106. Sinciput not so prominent	107. Sinciput Occiput not felt	108. Head on pelvic floor
Brim					

4 Puerperium

SHORT ANSWER QUESTIONS

Write short answers to the following.

1 Describe briefly the processes involved in the involution of the uterus.

2 Describe the physiology and purpose of the let-down reflex related to breastfeeding.

3 Describe the initiation of lactation and its continued regulation.

4 Identify and describe the three types of lochia following birth.

5 Describe the normalising of the cardiovascular system to a non-pregnant state following birth.

6 Describe the essential criteria/features of LAM to be an effective contraceptive.

7 Discuss the physiology related to hormonal contraception.

8 Describe the normalising of the urinary system to a non-pregnant state following birth.

9 Describe the return of the menstrual cycle following birth.

10 Describe how the musculoskeletal system returns to a non-pregnant state following birth.

TRUE OR FALSE?

Are the following statements true or false?

11 The intrauterine contraceptive device prevents implantation.

12 The ribcage always returns to a non-pregnant state following birth.

13 The external cervical os returns to a circular shape during the puerperium.

14 There is marked diuresis 48–72 hours following birth.

15 A fall in oxytocin levels following birth enables prolactin to produce milk.

16 Following birth, progesterone levels return to normal within 14 days.

17 Following birth, oestrogen levels return to normal within 7 days.

18 Women are more likely to experience coagulation difficulties postnatally.

19 If monitoring postnatal haemoglobin levels, venepuncture should occur on the third day.

20 The uterus remains an abdominal organ following the puerperium.

MULTIPLE CHOICE

Identify one correct answer for each of the following.

21 How much protection from pregnancy is afforded if the Bellagio consensus criteria for lactational amenorrhoea (LAM) are applied to contraception?

a) 20%

b) 50%

c) 98%

d) 75%

22 During breastfeeding, high levels of prolactin keep which hormone in abeyance, preventing return of the menstrual cycle?

a) thyroid stimulating hormone

b) follicle stimulating hormone

c) progesterone

d) oestrogen

23 How long do the effects of progesterone on muscles and ligaments last following birth?

a) 2–4 weeks

b) 3–5 days

c) 4–6 months

d) 1 year

24 Stress and anxiety in the puerperal period may delay any wound or tissue healing. This is due to the increased circulation of which hormone?

a) antidiuretic hormone

b) thyroxine

c) cortisol

d) renin

25 Following a second degree tear, healing of the perineum will involve which muscles?

a) transverse perineii

b) bulbocavernosus

c) sacrococcygeus

d) ileococcygeus

26 Maintenance of breastfeeding relies on which physiological response?

a) let-down

b) autocrine

c) endocrine

d) paracrine

27 Which protein is crucial in the maintenance of lactation?

a) oxytocin

b) prolactin

c) feedback inhibitor of lactation

d) prolactin inhibitor

28 The puerperium lasts for approximately how long?

a) 3 days

b) 6 weeks

c) 3 months

d) 10 days

29 Lochia is not described as?

a) rubra

b) serosa

c) alba

d) blanca

30 Which of the following is only found in lochia rubra?

a) erythrocytes

b) cervical mucus

c) bacteria

d) lanugo

31 Which hormone is responsible for after pains?

a) oxytocin

b) oestrogen

c) relaxin

d) progesterone

32 Which of the following is responsible for nipple trauma?

a) the use of nipple shields

b) effective attachment

c) frequent suckling

d) ineffective attachment

33 Which of the following contraceptive methods would not be recommended for a lactating mother?

a) combined oral contraceptive pill

b) progesterone only pill

c) Mirena intrauterine device

d) Depo-Provera injection

34 Within how many days would the uterus return to a pelvic organ?

a) 14 days

b) 3 days

c) 10 days

d) 28 days

35 Why is the postnatal woman at increased risk of thromboembolism?

a) postnatal diuresis

b) raised prolactin levels

c) increase in clotting factors

d) increase in white cells

FILL IN THE BLANKS

Fill in the blanks in each statement using the options in the box.

evaporation	above
alba	conduction
midway	odourless
no swelling	rubra
afterpains	baby blues
11	13
diuresis	increased lochia
convection	degradation of suture materials
venous engorgement	serosa
pain free	radiation

36 Immediately after birth the fundus of the uterus can be palpated _____ between the umbilicus and the symphysis pubis.

37 The day following normal birth the fundus of the uterus can be palpated _____ the level of the umbilicus.

38 Heat loss from the newborn baby can occur as a result of the following four processes: _____, _____, _____ and _____.

39 During the puerperium the maternal haemoglobin level returns to its normal range of _____ to _____ g/dl.

40 Vaginal loss following birth is known as lochia and occurs in three forms: _____, _____ and _____.

41 Within 24 hours of birth women are expected to lose fluid through the process of _____.

42 Women at 3 days post-birth are often said to be experiencing the following psychological phenomenon: _____ _____.

43 The four signs of healing a midwife would notice when inspecting the perineum on day 10 are: _____, _____, _____ and _____.

44 By the third postnatal day women will experience _____ _____ of the breast, irrespective of the feeding method chosen.

45 Effective breastfeeding in a multiparous woman can cause _____ _____ from the uterus and _____ of the uterus as a result of oxytocin release.

LABELLING EXERCISE

46–53 Figure 4.1 The prolactin response

Figure 4.2 The oxytocin reflex

Label the following diagrams: prolactin neurohormonal reflex, the oxytocic neurohormonal reflex (let-down reflex).

Baby suckles

Acini (milk-secreting) cells produce milk

Sensory impulses pass from the nipple to the brain

Oxytocin secreted by pituitary gland goes via bloodstream to the breasts

Baby suckles

Myoepithelial (muscle) cells contract and expel milk

Sensory impulses pass from the nipple to the brain

Prolactin secreted by pituitary gland goes via bloodstream to the breasts

---

Figure 4.1

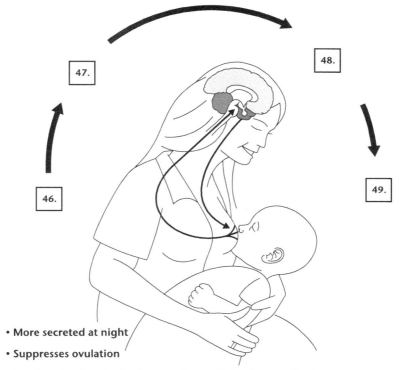

- More secreted at night
- Suppresses ovulation
- Level peaks after the feed, to produce milk for the next feed

Figure 4.2

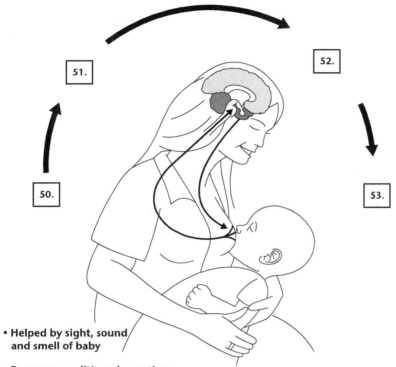

- Helped by sight, sound and smell of baby
- Becomes conditioned over time
- Hindered by anxiety, stress, pain and doubt
- Works before or during the feed to make the milk flow

ANSWERS

SHORT ANSWER QUESTIONS

1 **Describe briefly the processes involved in the involution of the uterus.**

Three processes are involved in the involution of the uterus: ischaemia, autolysis and phagocytosis. Following the separation of the placenta and action of the oblique muscles in the myometrium the blood supply is reduced causing death of the cells. These are subsequently broken down through autolysis using proteolytic enzymes to reduce the size of the cells. Lastly phagocytes remove the waste products via the blood and lymphatic systems.

2 **Describe the physiology and purpose of the let-down reflex related to breast feeding.**

The let-down or oxytocic reflex is neurohormonal. It is neuronally stimulated through the sight, smell, touch or cry of the baby, transmitting the message to the posterior pituitary gland stimulating the release of oxytocin. This travels through the bloodstream to act on smooth muscle within the myoepithelial cells of the breast to drive milk from the acini cells and along the lactiferous ducts towards the nipple openings.

3 **Describe the initiation of lactation and its continued regulation.**

Lactation is initiated following the birth of the baby and placenta. It is activated by the baby suckling effectively at the breast and is another neurohormonal reflex. The suckling baby stimulates a neural response to the anterior pituitary gland releasing prolactin, which is transported via the bloodstream. Prolactin receptors present on acini cells are subsequently activated and stimulate the acini cells to commence the secretion of milk. Inactivated prolactin receptor sites will shut down if not activated adequately soon after birth. Maintenance of lactation is mainly dependent on the balance of prolactin and the presence of feedback inhibitor of lactation (FIL), a protein found in breastmilk. The higher the level of FIL within the breast the greater the inhibitory effect – effective removal of milk is therefore essential to the maintenance of lactation. This is an autocrine response as it affects only one breast at a time. Remaining products of the third stage within the uterus will inhibit this process.

4 **Identify and describe the three types of lochia following birth.**

Lochia is the name given to vaginal loss which occurs following birth.

Rubra (red), occurring on day 1–3. This contains predominantly blood products especially erythrocytes, decidual cells, lanugo, vernix, meconium, amnion and chorion. Serosa (pink), occurring on days 4–10. This contains predominantly serum from blood, cervical discharge, microorganisms, degenerating deciduas. Alba (white/creamy), occurring on days 11–28. This contains leucocytes, decidual cells, mucus, bacteria and epithelial cells.

Vaginal loss during this period can be varied in duration, amount and colour. Most important is the sequential progression from rubra to alba. Any reversal of the process or offensive lochia needs investigating.

5 **Describe the normalising of the cardiovascular system to a non-pregnant state following birth.**

The increase in blood volume and haemodilution is reversed following the removal of oestrogen with the delivery of the placenta causing a diuresis within the first 48 hours. Plasma volume and haematocrit return to normal. Excess tissue fluid following the reduction in progesterone is removed and a return to normal vascular tone occurs. An increase in atrial natriuretic peptide (ANP) may contribute to the diuresis.

6 **Describe the essential criteria/features of LAM to be an effective contraceptive.**

The Bellagio consensus statement identified three factors which have to be in place for LAM to be an effective contraception and offer 98% protection. Firstly the woman must be amenorrhoeic since the birth of the baby. Secondly, she must be fully breastfeeding regularly throughout the day and night as the high level of circulating prolactin inhibits the release of gonadatrophin releasing hormone from the anterior pituitary gland thus preventing ovulation. Thirdly, the baby should be less than 6 months old.

7 **Discuss the physiology related to hormonal contraception.**

Synthetic oestrogens and progesterones are found in oral contraceptives. The oestrogen component inhibits FSH release stopping maturation of the follicle and progesterone inhibits LH stopping ovulation. Within a combined oral contraception the oestrogen component is constant but the progesterone component varies. This causes thickening of the mucus making implantation unsuitable and reduces the motility in the uterine tubes. A progesterone only contraceptive would be given to a lactating woman but a combined contraceptive could be prescribed for a formula feeding mother.

8 Describe the normalising of the urinary system to a non-pregnant state following birth.

During pregnancy there is increased excretion of fluid and breakdown products of protein by the kidneys. Reduction of progesterone following the removal of the placenta reduces the dilatation of the renal tract and renal organs return to their pre-pregnant state. Displacement of the bladder and urethra may cause difficulties with tone and micturition.

9 Describe the return of the menstrual cycle following birth.

Oestrogen levels return to the pre-pregnant levels by day 7 following removal of the placenta. Progesterone levels return to those of the luteal phase of the menstrual cycle by 24–48 hours and the follicular phase by day 7. Infertility following birth is common in the postnatal period particularly during lactation. Ovulation follows a rise in progesterone level, and is often anovulatory particularly in lactating women, but ovulation occurs in 25% of women, when pregnancy could occur.

10 Describe how the musculoskeletal system returns to a non-pregnant state following birth.

Progesterone and relaxin, which are high in pregnancy, drop following the delivery of the placenta. This therefore increases the tone in all smooth muscle, ligaments and joints. The sacroiliac and symphysis pubis joints are particularly susceptible to this change.

TRUE OR FALSE?

| 11 | The intrauterine contraceptive device prevents implantation. | ✔ |

| 12 | The ribcage always returns to a non-pregnant state following birth. | ✘ |

In most women the ribs remain flared following childbirth.

| 13 | The external cervical os returns to a circular shape during the puerperium. | ✘ |

The external cervical os forms a slit shape during the puerperium.

| 14 | There is marked diuresis 48–72 hours following birth. | ✔ |

| 15 | A fall in oxytocin levels following birth enables prolactin to produce milk. | ✘ |

A fall in progesterone levels following birth enables prolactin to produce milk.

| 16 | Following birth, progesterone levels return to normal within 14 days. | ✘ |

Following birth, progesterone levels return to normal within 7 days.

| 17 | Following birth, oestrogen levels return to normal within 7 days. | ✔ |

| 18 | Women are more likely to experience coagulation difficulties postnatally. | ✔ |

| 19 | If monitoring postnatal haemoglobin levels, venepuncture should occur on the third day. | ✔ |

| 20 | The uterus remains an abdominal organ following the puerperium. | ✘ |

By the end of the puerperium the uterus returns to being a pelvic organ.

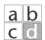 **MULTIPLE CHOICE ANSWERS**

Correct answers are in bold italics

21 How much protection from pregnancy is afforded if the Bellagio consensus criteria for lactational amenorrhoea (LAM) are applied to contraception?

a) 20%   b) 50%   *c) 98%*   d) 75%

22 During breastfeeding, high levels of prolactin keep which hormone in abeyance, preventing return of the menstrual cycle?

a) thyroid stimulating hormone   *b) follicle stimulating hormone*   c) progesterone
d) oestrogen

23 How long do the effects of progesterone on muscles and ligaments last following birth?

a) 2–4 weeks   b) 3–5 days   *c) 4–6 months*   d) 1 year

24 Stress and anxiety in the puerperal period may delay any wound or tissue healing. This is due to the increased circulation of which hormone?

a) antidiuretic hormone   b) thyroxine   *c) cortisol*   d) renin

25 Following a second degree tear, healing of the perineum will involve which muscles?

a) transverse perineii   b) bulbocavernosus   c) sacrococcygeus
d) ileococcygeus

26 Maintenance of breastfeeding relies on which physiological response?

a) let-down   *b) autocrine*   c) endocrine   d) paracrine

27 Which protein is crucial in the maintenance of lactation?

a) oxytocin   b) prolactin   *c) feedback inhibitor of lactation*   d) prolactin
inhibitor

28 The puerperium lasts for approximately how long?

a) 3 days   *b) 6 weeks*   c) 3 months   d) 10 days

29 Lochia is not described as?

a) rubra   b) serosa   c) alba   *d) blanca*

30 **Which of the following is only found in lochia rubra?**

a) erythrocytes   b) cervical mucus   c) bacteria   *d) lanugo*

31 **Which hormone is responsible for after pains?**

a) oxytocin   b) oestrogen   c) relaxin   d) progesterone

32 **Which of the following is responsible for nipple trauma?**

a) the use of nipple shields   b) effective attachment   c) frequent suckling
d) ineffective attachment

33 **Which of the following contraceptive methods would not be recommended for a lactating mother?**

a) combined oral contraceptive pill   b) progesterone only pill   c) Mirena intrauterine device   d) Depo-Provera injection

34 **Within how many days would the uterus return to a pelvic organ?**

a) 14 days   b) 3 days   *c) 10 days*   d) 28 days

35 **Why is the postnatal woman at increased risk of thromboembolism?**

a) postnatal diuresis   b) raised prolactin levels   *c) increase in clotting factors*
d) increase in white cells

FILL IN THE BLANKS

36 Immediately after birth the fundus of the uterus can be palpated *midway* between the umbilicus and the symphysis pubis.

37 The day following normal birth the fundus of the uterus can be palpated *above* the level of the umbilicus.

38 Heat loss from the newborn baby can occur as a result of the following four processes: *evaporation, conduction, convection* and *radiation*.

39 During the puerperium the maternal haemoglobin level returns to its normal range of *11* to *13* g/dl.

40 Vaginal loss following birth is known as lochia and occurs in three forms: *rubra, serosa* and *alba*.

41 Within 24 hours of birth women are expected to lose fluid through the process of *diuresis*.

42 Women at 3 days post-birth are often said to be experiencing the following psychological phenomenon: *baby blues*.

43 The four signs of healing a midwife would notice when inspecting the perineum on day 10 are: *pain free, no swelling, odourless* and *degradation of suture materials.*

44 By the third postnatal day women will experience *venous engorgement* of the breast, irrespective of the feeding method chosen.

45 Effective breastfeeding in a multiparous woman can cause *increased lochia* from the uterus and *afterpains* of the uterus as a result of oxytocin release.

LABELLING EXERCISE

Figure 4.1a

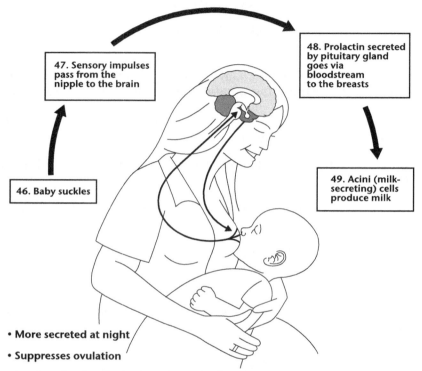

47. Sensory impulses pass from the nipple to the brain

48. Prolactin secreted by pituitary gland goes via bloodstream to the breasts

46. Baby suckles

49. Acini (milk-secreting) cells produce milk

• **More secreted at night**

• **Suppresses ovulation**

• **Level peaks after the feed, to produce milk for the next feed**

Figure 4.2a

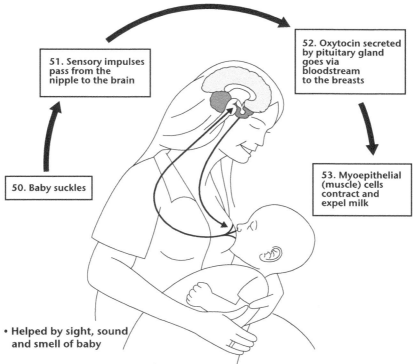

51. Sensory impulses pass from the nipple to the brain

52. Oxytocin secreted by pituitary gland goes via bloodstream to the breasts

50. Baby suckles

53. Myoepithelial (muscle) cells contract and expel milk

• Helped by sight, sound and smell of baby

• Becomes conditioned over time

• Hindered by anxiety, stress, pain and doubt

• Works before or during the feed to make the milk flow

PART 2
Pathophysiology

INTRODUCTION

Part 2 aims to allow readers to test their knowledge of the most common complications that present during pregnancy, the intrapartum and the postnatal periods.

Maternal mortality and morbidity from these complications remain a significant feature of care during these periods. It is essential therefore for students to develop a good understanding of the related pathophysiology.

It is impossible to provide questions for all diseases or complications. The approach adopted is to present a variety of questions to enable students to identify their learning needs and focus on their strengths and weaknesses to assist with their progress.

Although some of the short answers may involve reference to management of care, the main focus is on the pathophysiology related to the complications.

It is expected that students will consider the main principles of management within their own practice. This should include the process of assessment, implementation and evaluation of care, risk assessment, SBAR, MEOWS, close monitoring of basic observations to include respiration, temperature, pulse and blood pressure, ABC resuscitation, fetal well-being and haemodynamic monitoring with due consideration to evidence/research, the role of the midwife, multiprofessional teamwork, psychological, ethical and social aspects.

In the final chapters of Part 2 we deal with pharmacology and numeracy.

Useful resources:

Critical Care in Childbearing for Midwives. Mary Billington and Mandy Stevenson. Blackwell Publishing, 2007.

The Midwives' Guide to Key Medical Conditions: Pregnancy and Childbirth. Linda Wylie and Helen Bryce. Churchill Livingstone, Elsevier, 2008.

www.nice.org.uk

www.rcog.org.uk

www.rcoa.ac.uk

5 Pregnancy

SHORT ANSWER QUESTIONS

Write short answers to the following.

1. Describe the different types of anaemia in pregnancy.

2. Discuss the pathophysiology of a venous thromboembolic event.

3. What is gestational diabetes? List the risk factors and potential complications for mother and baby.

4. Describe the pathophysiology of sickle cell disease.

5. Outline the two main types of epileptic seizures.

6. Define the types of placenta praevia.

7. Describe the pathophysiology of a placental abruption.

8. What is pre-eclampsia? Outline the causes and risks to the mother and fetus.

9. What are the potential effects for mother and baby of group B streptococcus infection in pregnancy?

10. What is cholestasis? Outline the risks to the mother and fetus.

TRUE OR FALSE?

Are the following statements true or false?

11 Von Willebrand's disease is an autosomal dominant condition.

12 Hyperemesis is a risk factor for a venous thromboembolic event.

13 Thalassaemia is an autosomal dominant disorder.

14 Disseminated intravascular coagulation is a primary disease.

15 The term 'miscarriage' is defined as expulsion of the fetus by 12 weeks of pregnancy.

16 Gestational hypertension presents in the first and second trimesters of pregnancy.

17 Recommended treatment for eclampsia includes administration of magnesium sulphate.

18 Jaundice may be a sign of obstetric cholestasis.

19 Hydatidiform mole is characterised by decreasing levels of human chorionic gonatrophin until 10 weeks of pregnancy.

20 *Chlamydia trachomatis* is a common viral infection in women under 25 years of age.

MULTIPLE CHOICE

Identify one correct answer for each of the following.

21 At what level of bacteria count is asymptomatic bacteriuria established?

a) >1000 bacteria/ml of urine

b) >10,000 bacteria/ml of urine

c) >100,000 bacteria/ml of urine

d) >1,000,000 bacteria/ml of urine

22 Marfan's syndrome is caused by a defect on the chromosome:

a) 11

b) 16

c) 15

d) 9

23 *Treponema pallidum* is the causative organism for which one of the following?

a) genital warts

b) cytomegalovirus

c) conjunctivitis

d) syphilis

24 Endocarditis is:

a) stenosis of the cardiac valves

b) inflammation of the heart valves

c) ventricular septal defect

d) ischaemia of the heart valves

25 Beta thalassaemia major has:

a) 1 defective beta chain

b) 2 defective beta chains

c) 3 defective beta chains

d) 2 defective alpha chains

26 Glycosylated haemoglobin is used as an indicator of:

a) serum ferritin levels

b) mean cell volume

c) the level of glucose attached to haemoglobin a

d) serum blood glucose

27 CMV in pregnancy can lead to:

a) epilepsy in the neonate

b) maternal generalised oedema

c) a maternal rash

d) maternal constipation

28 In pregnancies complicated by hypothyroidism the demand for thyroxine increases by:

a) 5–10%

b) 10–20%

c) 25–50%

d) 60–90%

29 Pseudocyesis is:

a) excessive vomiting in pregnancy

b) excessive thirst in pregnancy

c) a skin rash in pregnancy

d) a phantom pregnancy

30 A grade two placenta praevia is defined as:

a) the placenta encroaches on the lower segment

b) the placenta fully covers the cervical os

c) the placenta reaches the internal cervical os

d) the placenta is in the lower segment of the uterus

31 A missed miscarriage is when:

a) the pregnancy is non-viable and products of conception remain in utero

b) the products of conception develop outside the uterine cavity

c) there is vaginal bleeding and abdominal pain with a viable fetus

d) some part of products is contained with heavy bleeding

32 Which one of the following pathophysiological changes does NOT occur with pre-eclampsia:

a) retinal arteriolar spasms

b) glomerular endothelial damage

c) hepatic ischaemia

d) thrombocytopenia

33 Symptoms of systemic lupus erythematosus often:

a) remain the same in pregnancy

b) decrease in pregnancy

c) worsen in pregnancy

d) completely disappear in pregnancy

34 Women suffering from iron deficiency anaemia are advised to avoid:

a) vitamin C

b) caffeine

c) moderate exercise

d) white bread

35 A Couvelaire uterus

a) occurs after a postpartum haemorrhage

b) occurs as a result of a placenta accreta

c) occurs as a result of a placental abruption

d) occurs as a result of placenta praevia

FILL IN THE BLANKS

Fill in the blanks in each statement using the options in the box

40	serum ferritin
pain	varicella zoster
24th	transplacental
(CD4) T-lymphocytes	inflammation
Africa	toxoplasmosis
swelling	haemolysis
elevated liver enzymers	platelets
West Indies	

36 An antepartum haemorrhage is defined as bleeding from the genital tract after the _____ week of gestation.

37 HIV usually infects the _____ cells of the immune system.

38 Morbid obesity is defined as a BMI of greater than _____.

39 Total iron body stores can be estimated by measuring _____ _____ levels.

40 Infection of a fetus in pregnancy from *Listeria monocytogenes* is by the _____ route.

41 Sickle cell disorders are most commonly found in women with origins from _____ or the _____ _____.

42 A protozoan parasitic infection that can cause miscarriage in pregnancy is known as _____.

43 Chicken pox is caused by the _____ _____virus.

44 The acronym 'H E L L P' stands for _____, _____ _____ _____ and low _____.

45 Symptoms of a deep vein thrombosis include: _____ and _____ in the area of the clot.

ANSWERS

SHORT ANSWER QUESTIONS

1 **Describe the different types of anaemia in pregnancy.**

Anaemia in pregnancy can be described as physiological, iron deficiency, folic acid deficiency or vitamin B_{12} deficiency. Physiological anaemia is caused by a maternal physiological increase in blood plasma volume, thus diluting the circulating red cell volume and causing haemodilution.

Iron deficiency anaemia is characterised by low haemoglobin, but this factor alone is not an indicator of the cause. Diagnosis of iron deficiency anaemia is by obtaining the mean cell volume (MCV) and the mean cell haemoglobin concentration (MCHC) levels in blood. These indicate the average volume occupied by a red cell and the concentration of haemoglobin within a red blood cell in the circulation. Therefore iron deficiency anaemia is described as microcytic and hypochromic. Further haematological testing for serum iron levels, total iron binding capacity will reveal the level of iron stored in the tissues; and serum ferritin levels will demonstrate total body stores of iron.

Folic acid demand is increased in pregnancy as it is needed for cell growth and there is a physiological decrease in serum folate levels. A reduced intake of folic acid or impairment of absorption will result in red cells that are reduced in number but have a larger size, leading to a macrocytic or megoblastic anaemia with the MCV rising, the MCHC staying the same and the haemoglobin level falling. Signs and symptoms of folic acid deficiency anaemia include weight loss, nausea and vomiting, and diarrhoea.

Vitamin B_{12} deficiency also results in megoblastic anaemia and is most likely to be seen in women whose Vitamin B_{12} intake is reduced. Vitamin B_{12} is needed for normal functioning of the brain and nervous system and for the formation of blood. Vitamin B_{12} is predominantly found in animal and dairy products, therefore pregnant women who are vegan will need to take supplements.

2 **Discuss the pathophysiology of a venous thromboembolic event.**

A venous thromboembolic event is a generalised term that can be used to describe either a deep vein thrombosis or a pulmonary embolism. In pregnancy women are more susceptible to this condition due to hypercoagulation, stasis of blood flow and endothelial injury to blood vessels – these three elements are known as Virchow's triad. As part of pregnancy, coagulation factors increase in readiness for labour, plus a woman may have an underlying thrombophilia such as factor V Leiden. Pressure on the inferior vena cava and the pelvic veins by the gravid uterus contributes to stasis of blood flow and inflammatory changes in the veins can cause changes to the vessel wall leading to deposition of platelets. A thrombus is formed in a deep vein which partially or completely occludes blood flow through that vein. A part of the thrombus can break off and travel through the right side of the heart into the pulmonary arterial system causing a pulmonary embolus.

3 **What is gestational diabetes? List the risk factors and potential complications for mother and baby.**

Gestational diabetes is an impaired glucose tolerance during pregnancy. During pregnancy the placenta secretes substances that have an anti-insulin effect; if the beta islet cells are unable to produce more insulin to counteract this effect then gestational diabetes will follow. It is usually asypmtomatic and is diagnosed by haematological screening – a glucose tolerance test – due to identified risk factors such as previous gestational diabetes, previous macrosomic baby, previous stillbirth, a family history of diabetes, maternal obesity and polyhydramnios. It may cause or contribute towards macrosomia, polyhydramnios, premature labour, pre-eclampsia or intra-uterine growth restriction. Women may develop gestational diabetes again in subsequent pregnancies or may develop type 2 diabetes. They are at increased risk of developing type 2 diabetes in later life. Potential complications for the fetus/neonate include birth asphyxia if shoulder dystocia occurs, hepatomegaly, polycythyaemia, I U F D or neonatal hypoglycaemia.

4 **Describe the pathophysiology of sickle cell disease.**

Sickle cell disease is an autosomal recessive disorder in which affected individuals are homozygous. Individuals who have sickle cell trait are heterozygous: an abnormal gene must be inherited from each parent for sickle cell disease to occur. Sickle cell disease is caused by an abnormality in the formation and quality of the adult haemoglobin molecule. Normally blood cells have four pairs of globin chains, one pair of alpha and a pair of beta chains. In affected individuals the amino acid glutamic acid is substituted for either valine or lysine on the beta chain. This results in the membranes of the red cells becoming fragile. They have a reduced life span of approximately 10–20 days causing chronic haemolytic anaemia. During deoxygenation these cells become crystallised and distorted. These erythrocytes become sickle shaped and are easily haemolysed. Certain conditions such as hypoxia or infection cause agglutination of these sickle cells leading to blockage of blood capillaries and subsequent ischaemia of the surrounding tissues. This is known as a sickle cell crisis.

5 **Outline the two main types of epileptic seizures.**

Epileptic seizures are known to have over 40 categories but there are two main types, partial seizures and generalised seizures.

Partial seizures can be either simple or complex, and are often preceded by an 'aura', a feeling of light-headedness and/or dizziness, intense feelings of discomfort or foreboding, altered vision and hearing. It originates from either the frontal or temporal lobe of the brain and may extend to a generalised seizure. During a simple partial seizure the woman remains fully conscious throughout and may experience symptoms such as changes in the way things look, feel, or smell, a feeling of *déjà vu*, tingling or muscle stiffness in the limbs, intense emotions or twitching on one side of the body. A complex partial seizure involves unusual body behaviour such as lip smacking, hand rubbing, fiddling with objects or chewing or swallowing.

A generalised seizure can be subdivided further into six main types and may be preceded by an aura. These involve both hemispheres of the brain. An absence seizure (petit mal) is seen mainly in children; usually the child loses awareness of their surroundings for about 20 seconds and will have no memory of the seizure. Myoclonic jerks cause the limbs to briefly twitch with no loss of consciousness. A clonic seizure causes similar twitching to that of myoclonic jerks except that the symptoms may last up to two minutes with loss of consciousness. An atonic seizure causes all muscles to relax; conversely a tonic seizure causes all muscles to suddenly become stiff. The most common type of seizure is a tonic-clonic seizure (grand mal) which is characterised by possibly an aura, sudden stiffness of the limbs followed by twitching of the limbs, often with unconsciousness.

6 **Define the types of placenta praevia.**

A placenta praevia is an abnormally situated placenta, wholly or partly in the lower uterine segment. It can be classified by the location of the placenta in relation to the uterus. A type I placenta praevia is found mainly in the upper segment but encroaches on the lower segment. A type II placenta praevia reaches to, but does not cover, the internal cervical os. A type III placenta praevia covers the cervical internal os when it is closed but not completely when it is dilated. A type IV placenta praevia completely covers the internal cervical os. Placenta praevia may also be described as a major praevia if it lies wholly over the cervical os and a minor or partial praevia if it lies in the lower segment but is not covering the cervical os.

7 **Describe the pathophysiology of a placental abruption.**

A placental abruption is defined as premature separation of a normally situated placenta, causing blood loss from the mother that may be concealed, revealed, or revealed and concealed (mixed). As separation ensues the maternal venous sinuses in the placental bed bleed. If blood escapes from the central site it causes separation of that part of the placenta from the uterine wall and the formation of a blood clot that pushes the placenta away from the uterine wall with little or no visible blood loss. This is known as a concealed abruption. If the separation occurs from the placental edge blood seeps out from the side of the membranes down the uterine wall to drain out through the vagina – this is known as a revealed abruption. A mixture of both types is also common. A further complication is when blood retained in the uterus may subsequently be forced into the myometrial fibres causing bruising and irritability to the fibres – this is known as a Couvelaire uterus.

8 **What is pre-eclampsia? Outline the causes and risks to the mother and fetus.**

Pre-eclampsia is a multi-factorial condition of pregnancy characterised by raised blood pressure and significant proteinurea occurring after 20 weeks of pregnancy. This can present with signs and symptoms such as headache, blurred vision, abdominal or epigastric pain, and deranged haemotological biochemistry including low platelets and abnormal liver enzymes. It can lead to the convulsive condition known as eclampsia. As a hypertensive disease of pregnancy it represents a significant cause of maternal and fetal mortality and morbidity.

It is thought that the secondary invasion of maternal spiral arteries by trophoblasts in the placenta is impaired subsequently leading to decreased placental function. Due to these hypoxic placental changes endothelial cells secrete fewer vasodilators and platelets secrete more thrombexane. This leads to generalised vasoconstriction and decreased aldosterone secretion. This in turn leads to vasospasm and raised maternal blood pressure. Continued hypertension leads to trophoblastic cell injury; fragments are released and are carried to the lungs where they are destroyed, which causes the release of thromboplastins subsequently causing intravascular coagulation and thrombosis. This also leads to fibrin deposition in the kidneys which reduces the glomerular filtration rate and increases the permeability of the endothelial tissue resulting in proteinuria and hypovolaemia. Fibrin deposition in the central nervous system will cause convulsions.

Risks to the mother include intracranial haemorrhage, encephalopathy, placental abruption, retinal detachment and renal failure. Risks to the fetus are due to placental insufficiency and include preterm labour, intrauterine growth restriction and stillbirth.

9 | **What are the potential effects for mother and baby of group B streptococcus infection in pregnancy?**

Group B streptococcus (GBS) is a gram positive bacterium that naturally colonises both men and women and usually causes no symptoms to carriers. It is usually found in the gastrointestinal tract, may be found in the back of the throat and also the vagina and it is often an intermittent colonisation. In pregnancy the risks are to the fetus through vertical transmission as the bacteria are able to infiltrate the amniotic cavity to infect the fetus via the lung epithelium. A baby born with a GBS infection in the early days of life may have septicaemia, meningitis or pneumonia; GBS infection in the early neonatal period causes the deaths of approximately 75 babies per annum in the UK. Babies who develop meningitis due to GBS and survive may have morbidity issues such as learning difficulties, impaired sight or hearing and lung damage. Late onset GBS infection in babies occurring after 7 days may present with meningitis and septicaemia and can be transmitted through the skin and the respiratory tract of carriers.

10 | **What is cholestasis? Outline the risks to the mother and fetus.**

Cholestasis, also known as intrahepatic cholestasis of pregnancy, is a multifactorial condition in pregnancy characterised by pruritus (itching, commonly on the palms of the hands and soles of the feet) without a skin rash and abnormal haematological liver function tests. Bile acids may also be raised. The itching, the abnormal liver function tests and bile acids should resolve once the baby is born. It is important when managing the disease to exclude other potential causes of pruritus and abnormal LFTs.

The incidence of intrahepatic cholestasis of pregnancy is influenced by environmental and genetic factors and varies worldwide. Women are more at risk of a postpartum haemorrhage; there is an increased risk of preterm birth (both spontaneous and iatrogenic) and a debatable increased risk of stillbirth.

TRUE OR FALSE?

11 **Von Willebrand's disease is an autosomal dominant condition.**

12 **Hyperemesis is a risk factor for a venous thromboembolic event.**

13 **Thalassaemia is an autosomal dominant disorder.**

Thalassaemia is an autosomal recessive disorder.

14 **Disseminated intravascular coagulation is a primary disease.**

Disseminated intravascular coagulation is a secondary disorder that occurs in response to a number of diseases or disorders.

15 **The term 'miscarriage' is defined as expulsion of the fetus by 12 weeks of pregnancy.**

The term 'miscarriage' refers to the expulsion of the fetus up to 23+6 weeks of pregnancy. Three quarters of all miscarriages occur in the first 12 weeks of pregnancy.

16 **Gestational hypertension presents in the first and second trimesters of pregnancy.**

17 **Recommended treatment for eclampsia includes administration of magnesium sulphate.**

18 **Jaundice may be a sign of obstetric cholestasis.**

19 **Hydatidiform mole is characterised by deceasing levels of human chorionic gonatrophin until 10 weeks of pregnancy.**

Hydatidiform mole is characterised by elevated levels of human chorionic gonadatrophin levels until 10 weeks of pregnancy.

20 ***Chlamydia trachomatis* is a common viral infection in women under 25 years of age.**

Chlamydia trachomatis is a bacterial infection. It can be contracted by both men and women; it is common in woman under 25 years of age.

MULTIPLE CHOICE

Correct answers identified in bold italics

21 **Asymptomatic bacteriuria is when the bacteria count is:**

a) >1000 bacteria/ml of urine   b) >10,000 bacteria/ml of urine   *c) >100,000 bacteria/ml of urine*   d) >1,000,000 bacteria/ml of urine

Asymptomatic bacteriuria occurs in 5–7% of pregnant women and if left untreated may lead to pyelonephritis.

22 **Marfan's syndrome is caused by a defect on the chromosome:**

a) 11   b) 16   *c) 15*   d) 9

23 ***Treponema pallidum* is the causative organism for:**

a) genital warts   b) cytomegalovirus   c) conjunctivitis   *d) syphilis*

24 **Endocarditis is:**

a) stenosis of the cardiac valves   *b) inflammation of the heart valves*
c) ventricular septal defect   d) ischaemia of the heart valves

25 **Beta thalassaemia major has:**

a) 1 defective beta chain   *b) 2 defective beta chains*   c) 3 defective beta chains
d) 2 defective alpha chains

26 **Glycosylated haemoglobin is used as an indicator of:**

a) serum ferritin levels   b) mean cell volume   *c) the level of glucose attached to haemoglobin a*   d) serum blood glucose

27 **CMV in pregnancy can lead to:**

a) epilepsy in the neonate   b) maternal generalised oedema   c) a maternal rash   d) maternal constipation

28 **In pregnancies complicated by hypothyroidism the demand for thyroxine increases by:**

a) 5–10%   b) 10–20%   *c) 25–50%*   d) 69–90%

29 Pseudocyesis is:

a) excessive vomiting in pregnancy   b) excessive thirst in pregnancy   c) a skin rash in pregnancy   *d) a phantom pregnancy*

30 A grade two placenta praevia is defined as:

a) the placenta encroaches on the lower segment   b) the placenta fully covers the cervical os   c) the placenta reaches the internal cervical os   *d) the placenta is in the lower segment of the uterus*

31 A missed miscarriage is when:

a) the pregnancy is non-viable and products of conception remain in utero

b) the products of conception develop outside the uterine cavity

c) there is vaginal bleeding and abdominal pain with a viable fetus

d) some part of the product of conception is contained with heavy bleeding

32 Which one of the following pathophysiological changes do NOT occur with pre-eclampsia:

a) retinal arteriolar spasms   b) glomerular endothelial damage   c) hepatic ischaemia   *d) thrombocytopenia*

33 Symptoms of systemic lupus erythematosus often:

a) remain the same in pregnancy   b) decrease in pregnancy   *c) worsen in pregnancy*   d) completely disappear in pregnancy

34 Women suffering from iron deficiency anaemia are advised to avoid:

a) vitamin C   *b) caffeine*   c) moderate exercise   d) white bread

35 A Couvelaire uterus

a) occurs after a postpartum haemorrhage   b) occurs as a result of a placenta accreta   *c) occurs as a result of a placental abruption*   d) occurs as a result of placenta praevia

FILL IN THE BLANKS

36 An antepartum haemorrhage is defined as bleeding from the genital tract after the *24th* week of gestation.

37 HIV usually infects the *(CD4) T-lymphocyte* cells of the immune system.

38 Morbid obesity is defined as a BMI of greater than *40*.

39 Total iron body stores can be estimated by measuring *serum ferritin* levels.

40 Infection of a fetus in pregnancy from *Listeria monocytogenes* is by the *transplacental* route.

41 Sickle cell disorders are most commonly found in women with origins from *Africa* or the *West Indies.*

42 A protozoan parasitic infection that can cause miscarriage in pregnancy is known as *toxoplasmosis.*

43 Chicken pox is caused by the *varicella zoster* virus.

44 The acronym 'HELLP' stands for *haemolysis, elevated liver enzymes* and low *platelets.*

45 Symptoms of a deep vein thrombosis include: *pain, inflammation* and *swelling* in the area of the clot.

6 Intrapartum

SHORT ANSWER QUESTIONS

Write short answers to the following.

1 Describe the main methods of induction of labour.

2 Outline the reasons for a cord prolapse.

3 Discuss the predisposing factors for a breech presentation.

4 Describe the mechanism of labour for an occipito-posterior presentation.

5 Identify the maternal and fetal risks associated with a multiple pregnancy.

6 Outline the predisposing factors associated with preterm labour.

7 Discuss the management of a retained placenta.

8 Describe the types of adherent placentae.

9 What is disseminated intravascular coagulation?

10 Outline the potential complications associated with epidural anaesthesia in labour.

TRUE OR FALSE?

Are the following statements true or false?

11 During an asthma attack cells are saturated with carbon dioxide.

12 An abruptio placenta is associated with painless bleeding.

13 A feature of disseminated intravascular coagulation is a decrease in fibrinogen.

14 An acute inversion of the uterus occurs after 48 hours following birth.

15 The Lovset manoeuvre is a recognised technique in the management of shoulder dystocia.

16 Complete rupture of the uterus involves a tear in the wall of the uterus with or without expulsion of the fetus.

17 The Mauriceau-Smellie-Veit manoeuvre consists of flexion and traction of the fetal head in a breech birth.

18 One of the signs of H E L L P is the development of hyperbilirubinaemia.

19 The engaging diameter in a face presentation in labour is submentovertical at 11.5 cm.

20 Amniotic fluid embolism is caused by amniotic fluid entering the maternal circulation via the placental sinuses.

MULTIPLE CHOICE

Identify one correct answer for each of the following.

21 The calculation of MAP reflects:

a) the mean pressure in the arterial system during one complete cycle

b) the mean venous pressure in the system during one complete cycle

c) the average diastolic pressure in the system during one complete cycle

d) the average systolic pressure in the system during one complete cycle

22 Intrapartum risk factors for shoulder dystocia include:

a) use of Syntocinon

b) precipitate labour

c) preterm labour

d) maternal semi-supine position in labour

23 Predisposing factors for spontaneous preterm labour include:

a) hypertension

b) herpes simplex virus

c) raised body mass index

d) epilepsy

24 Which of the following prerequisites is NOT required for a forceps birth?

a) bladder catheterisation

b) adequate maternal analgesia

c) a presenting part + 2 cm below the ischial spines

d) completely dilated cervix

25 Management of a cord prolapse includes:

a) continuous maternal oxygen via a face mask

b) application of a fetal scalp electrode

c) maternal bladder filling

d) placing the woman in the McRoberts position

26 Complications of epidural anaesthesia include:

a) total spinal block

b) diarrhoea

c) maternal hypertension

d) hyperventilation

27 A breech birth mechanism is when:

a) the denominator is the mentum

b) the position is left occipto-anterior

c) the mentum points to the left ilio-pectineal eminence

d) the bitrochanteric diameter enters the pelvis first

28 Placenta percreta is when:

a) the placenta invades the myometrium

b) the placenta is embedded in the decidua basalis

c) the placenta penetrates through the myometrium

d) the placenta is adherent to the myometrium

29 Obstructed labour is characterised by:

a) Bandl's ring

b) efficient uterine action

c) rapid cervical effacement and dilatation

d) mild abdominal pain

30 Primary postpartum haemorrhage is NOT caused by:

a) cervical lacerations

b) sepsis

c) atonic uterus

d) retained products of conception

FILL IN THE BLANKS

Fill in the blanks in each statement using the options in the box.

10%	help
monozygotic	respiratory
cord prolapse	pressure
roll over	vasodilatation
legs	episiotomy
enter	Mendelson's
unfavourable	remove posterior arm
fall	short
posterior	tone
1%	20%

31 The main four causes of a primary postpartum haemorrhage are _____ (70%), trauma (_____), tissue (_____), thrombin (_____).

32 Administration of local anaesthetic during epidural anaesthesia affects the sympathetic nervous system causing _____ and subsequent _____ in blood pressure.

33 H E L P E R R is a mnemonic for shoulder dystocia and stands for H_____, E_____, L_____, P_____, E_____, R_____, R_____.

34 A persistent occipito-posterior position results from a _____ rotation of the fetal occiput.

35 A vaginal birth is not possible in a persistent mento-_____ position.

36 If the placenta of a twin birth is monochorionic then the babies must be _____.

37 A modified Bishop's score of 2 indicates an _____cervix.

38 Cricoid pressure is applied during induction of general anaesthesia to help prevent _____ syndrome.

39 Exaggerated Simm's position is one of the maternal positions indicated when a _____ _____ is diagnosed.

40 A potential complication of epidural anaesthesia is a total spinal block leading to a _____ arrest.

ANSWERS

SHORT ANSWER QUESTIONS

1 **Describe the main methods of induction of labour.**

Induction of labour is started by artificial means from about 24 weeks gestation. The main methods are described as follows:

Membrane sweep: usually carried out after 40 weeks by a midwife or doctor. A digital vaginal examination is performed and the operator digitally separates the chorion from the cervix using a 360 degree circular action. It is suggested that the act of sweeping the membranes stimulates the production of natural prostaglandin production.

Artificial prostaglandin: artificial hormones are inserted into the body to replicate the naturally occurring prostaglandins. The aim is to stimulate cervical ripening; effacement and subsequent dilatation of the cervix by absorption into the tissues/epithelium of the vagina and cervix which then promotes uterine contractions. There are a number of preparations in use such as gels, pessaries, tablets and tampons placed in the posterior fornix of the vagina. Due to some of the potential risks associated with artificial prostaglandins such as hypertonicity, placental abruption, fetal hypoxia and amniotic fluid embolism, careful monitoring of maternal and fetal condition is required.

Artificial rupture of membranes (ARM) or amniotomy is performed when the cervix is assessed as favourable and the presenting part is engaged in the pelvis. This may precede the above methods or can be used independently. The membranes lying in front of the presenting part are ruptured using an amnihook to release the amniotic fluid. The loss is assessed for colour and amount.

Uterotonic drugs: Syntocinon is a strong synthetic agent used to stimulate the oxytocin receptors within the myometruim into action. It is commonly used for induction of labour after ARM and 6 hours after prostaglandin. The risks associated with its use are: uterine hyperstimulation and hypertony; uterine rupture; fetal hypoxia and asphyxia; fluid retention; postpartum haemorrhage; amniotic fluid embolism and operative or instrumental birth. Therefore it is essential that attention is paid to dosage and monitoring. It is administered by slow intravenous infusion using an infusion pump. The aim is to achieve effective regular contractions of 3–4 every 10 minutes, so the dose is titrated against uterine contractions.

2 | Outline the reasons for a cord prolapse.

Cord prolapse is where the cord escapes before the presenting part when the membranes have ruptured. This is an obstetric emergency and prompt management is required. A cord presentation whereby the cord is felt behind intact membranes may cause a subsequent cord prolapse if the membranes rupture. Spontaneous rupture of membranes and ARM especially with a high head and malpresentation predisposes to a cord prolapse as the cord is able to slip down in front of the presenting part. Polyhydramnios with subsequent rupture of membranes may also lead to a cord prolapse as the gush and force of liquor may cause the cord to slip out before the presenting part.

3 | Discuss the predisposing factors for a breech presentation.

Breech presentation is when the buttocks present in the lower pole of the uterus. The predisposing factors for a breech presentation are when the legs are extended and it is difficult for the fetus to resume a flexed position; if a baby is born before 35 weeks the fetus may present in a breech as it is easier for the fetus to move in utero; in multiple pregnancies there is limited space for the fetus to move, therefore the fetus may remain in a fixed position i.e. a breech; in cases of polyhydramnios the large amount of liquor may allow the fetus to be more mobile; hydrocephaly increases the size of the fetal head, it is therefore unable fit in the pelvis; uterine abnormalities such as fibroids or a bicornuate uterus or a low lying placenta may also prevent the fetal head entering the pelvis.

4 | Describe the mechanism of labour for an occipito-posterior presentation.

The occiput lies in the posterior aspect of the pelvis causing the head to be deflexed. There are two possible outcomes for the mechanism – a long or a short rotation. The mechanism of labour for a right occipito-posterior (ROP) position that take a long rotation is as follows: it is a longitudinal lie, vertex presentation with an attitude of a deflexed head. The denominator is the occiput with an occipitofrontal diameter of 11.5 cm which lies in the right oblique of the pelvic brim. The occiput becomes the leading part with descent and when it reaches the pelvic floor rotates forwards 1/8 of a circle along the right side of the pelvis to lie under the symphysis pubis. The shoulders follow to turn 2/8 circle to the right oblique diameter. The occiput than escapes under the symphysis and the head is crowned. The sinciput, face and chin are delivered and the head is born by extension. Restitution occurs when the fetal head rights itself with the shoulders so that the head and shoulder are in the same plane. The shoulders enter the pelvis in the right oblique diameter, the anterior shoulder reaches the pelvic floor to rotate forwards 1/8 of a circle to present under the symphysis pubis. This causes the occiput to rotate at the same time to the right. The anterior shoulder births under the symphysis pubis and the baby is born.

The other outcome occurs because the occiput fails to rotate forwards so the sinciput becomes the leading part and the occiput goes into the hollow of the sacrum to be born with the face towards the symphysis pubis; this is also known as 'face to pubis' or a 'short rotation' or a 'persistent occipito-posterior'.

5 | Identify the maternal and fetal risks associated with a multiple pregnancy.

The maternal and fetal risks factors associated with multiple pregnancy include an increase in the following: fetal abnormalities, preterm labour, anaemia, polyhydramnios, twin to twin transfusion, malpresentations, perinatal mortality and morbidity rates, IUGR, conjoined twins, premature rupture of membranes, prolapsed cord, prolonged labour, locked twins, delay in birth of second twin, postpartum haemorrhage and undiagnosed twins.

6 | Outline the predisposing factors associated with preterm labour.

Preterm labour is defined as occurring in the presence of uterine contractions which lead to effacement and dilatation of the cervix before 37 completed weeks of pregnancy. Although most causes are unknown, the main predisposing factors include cervical incompetence, antepartum haemorrhage, prelabour rupture of membranes, multiple pregnancy, fetal and maternal infections, smoking, maternal age over 35 years, hypertensive disorders of pregnancy, maternal diabetes, congenital abnormalities and rhesus incompatibility.

7 | Discuss the management of a retained placenta.

A retained or partially separated placenta prohibits good uterine contraction which may cause a postpartum haemorrhage. A retained placenta is when the placenta fails to deliver in the expected time interval of at least 1 hour (WHO) or 30 minutes despite active management of the third stage or 60 minutes with physiological management of the third stage of labour. If the placenta is trapped but detached, the use of controlled cord traction is recommended. If the uterus is atonic, the administration of a uterotonic drug may be considered but this can make manual removal more difficult due to constriction of the cervix. Other methods that may be considered are an injection of a uterotonic agent into the umbilical cord. As there is a high risk of PPH with a retained placenta, the midwife must consider the following management: bladder catheterisation, estimation of blood loss, medical assistance, maternal observations, intravenous infusion to maintain haemodynamic stability and effective analgesia. Administration of some or all of the above uterotonic drugs may be attempted prior to manual removal of retained placenta under effective anaesthesia. Prophylactic broad spectrum antibiotics are administered to reduce the risk of endometritis. A full aseptic technique in theatre is required which involves careful digital removal starting from the edge of the placenta. One hand follows the path of the cord to the lower uterine segment to find the maternal–placental interface, the other hand stabilises the uterine fundus abdominal and the internal hand gently peels the placenta away with the fingers. The midwife/obstetrician should be aware of the possibility of an adherent placenta which may lead on to a hysterectomy.

8 **Describe the types of adherent placentae.**

There are three types: placenta accreta whereby the chorionic villi adhere to the myometrium, placenta increta whereby the chorionic villi invade the myometrium and placenta percreta whereby the chorionic villi grow through the myometrium and may invade other organs such as the bladder or the rectum. The adherent placenta may be either partially adherent or totally adherent.

9 **What is disseminated intravascular coagulation?**

Disseminated intravascular coagulation (DIC) is when the normal clotting mechanism is disrupted and is usually triggered by maternal or fetal conditions such as IUFD, eclampsia, severe haemorrhage, sepsis, AFE and hypovolaemic shock. Widespread clotting occurs, which causes the production of microthrombi in the circulation; this causes an increase of clots in the microcirculation, in the large vessels and in the organs, which leads to ischaemia and impaired organ perfusion. The increased clotting releases thromboplastin causing fibrinolysis and the production of fibrin degradation products (FDPs) which have anticoagulant properties. This produces a feedback mechanism to correct the clots causing more haemorrhage. DIC is associated with a poor prognosis and high mortality.

10 **Outline the potential complications associated with epidural anaesthesia in labour.**

The potential complications with epidural anaesthesia include block failure when the pain relief is inadequate. Hypotension can be caused by the vasodilation of the vessels of the lower limbs due to the drugs administered during an epidural; to reduce the risk of this a pre-loading dose of 500 ml of a crystalloid can be administered. Treatment is by increasing the IV volume infused or, if severe, by administration of a sympathomimetic vasoconstrictor. Loss of sensation to the bladder may occur which may necessitate urinary catheterisation. Epidural toxicity is another problem that can occur and results in a cluster of symptoms from tingling around mouth, tinnitus, tremor, irritability, dizziness, blurred vision, seizures, drowsiness, loss of consciousness, and respiratory and cardiac arrest. Dural puncture or dural tap may occur when the dura is accidently punctured causing leakage of CSF into the dural space. The woman may then experience severe postdural puncture headaches. Another complication is a total block when the epidural spreads up to the lungs/chest causing paralysis of the intercostal muscles and diaphragm and loss of sympathetic function to the heart. This requires emergency treatment as it can lead to respiratory arrest.

TRUE OR FALSE?

11 **During an asthma attack cells are saturated with carbon dioxide.**

Body cells are deprived of oxygen and therefore CO_2 build-up can lead to respiratory acidosis.

12 **An abruptio placenta is associated with painless bleeding.**

Placental abruption is associated with painful bleeding.

13 **A feature of disseminated intravascular coagulation is a decrease in fibrinogen.**

Fibrinogen is required to produce fibrin and assists with the clotting mechanism.

14 **An acute inversion of the uterus occurs in after 48 hours following birth.**

An acute uterine inversion occurs in the first 24 hours after birth.

15 **The Lovset manoeuvre is a recognised technique in the management of shoulder dystocia.**

Lovset is a technique used in the removal of extended arms in a breech birth.

16 **Complete rupture of the uterus involves a tear in the wall of the uterus with or without expulsion of the fetus.**

17 **The Mauriceau-Smellie-Veit manoeuvre consists of flexion and traction of the fetal head in a breech birth.**

18 **One of the signs of HELLP is the development of hyperbilirubinaemia.**

Increased haemolysis prevents normal physiological processes to occur and raises the serum liver enzymes.

19 **The engaging diameter in a face presentation in labour is submentovertical at 11.5 cm.**

The engaging diameter is the submentobregmatic of 9.5 cm. The submentovertical is the diameter that sweeps the perineum.

20 **Amniotic fluid embolism is caused by amniotic fluid entering the maternal circulation via the placental sinuses.**

MULTIPLE CHOICE
Correct answers in bold italics

21 **The calculation of MAP reflects:**

a) the mean pressure in the arterial system during one complete cycle

b) the mean venous pressure in the system during one complete cycle

c) the average diastolic pressure in the system during one complete cycle

d) the average systolic pressure in the system during one complete cycle

22 **Intrapartum risk factors for shoulder dystocia include:**

a) use of Syntocinon   b) precipitate labour   c) preterm labour   d) maternal semi-supine position labour

23 **Predisposing factors for spontaneous preterm labour include:**

a) hypertension   b) herpes simplex virus   c) raised body mass index   d) epilepsy

24 **Which of the following prerequisites is NOT required for a forceps birth?**

a) bladder catheterisation   b) adequate maternal analgesia   *c) a presenting part +2 cm below the ischial spines*   d) completely dilated cervix

25 **Management of a cord prolapse includes:**

a) continuous maternal oxygen via a face mask   b) application of a fetal scalp electrode   *c) maternal bladder filling*   d) placing the woman in the McRoberts position

26 **Complications of epidural anaesthesia include:**

a) total spinal block   b) diarrhoea   c) maternal hypertension   d) hyperventilation

27 **A breech birth mechanism is when:**

a) the denominator is the mentum   b) the position is left occipito-anterior   c) the mentum points to the left ilio-pectineal eminence   *d) the bitrochanteric diameter enters the pelvis first*

28 **Placenta percreta is when:**

a) the placenta invades the myometrium   b) the placenta is embedded in the decidua basalis   *c) the placenta penetrates through the myometrium*   d) the placenta is adherent to the myometrium

29 **Obstructed labour is characterised by:**

a) Bandl's ring   b) efficient uterine action   c) rapid cervical effacement and dilatation   d) mild abdominal pain

30 **Primary postpartum haemorrhage is NOT caused by**

a) cervical lacerations   *b) sepsis*   c) atonic uterus   d) retained products of conception

FILL IN THE BLANKS

31 The main four causes of primary postpartum haemorrhage are *tone* (70%), trauma *(20%), tissue (10%),* thrombin *(1%)*.

32 Administration of local anaesthetic during epidural anaesthesia affects the sympathetic nervous system causing *vasodilatation* and subsequent *fall* in blood pressure.

33 **HELPERR** is a mnemonic for shoulder dystocia and stands for *Help, Episiotomy, Legs, Pressure, Enter, Remove posterior arm, Roll over.*

34 A persistent occipito-posterior position results from a *short* rotation of the fetal occiput.

35 A vaginal birth is not possible in a persistent mento-*posterior* position.

36 If the placenta of a twin birth is monochorionic then the babies must be *monozygotic.*

37 A modified Bishop's score of 2 indicates an *unfavourable* cervix.

38 Cricoid pressure is applied during induction of general anaesthesia to help prevent *Mendelson's* syndrome.

39 Exaggerated Simm's position is one of the maternal positions indicated when a *cord prolapse* is diagnosed.

40 A potential complication of epidural anaesthesia is a total spinal block leading to a *respiratory* arrest.

7 Puerperium

SHORT ANSWER QUESTIONS

Write short answers to the following.

1 Outline the common complications of the puerperium.

2 Discuss a management plan for a woman who is unable to pass urine postnatally.

3 What is a postdural puncture headache? Briefly outline the midwife's role in caring for a woman who is diagnosed with a postdural puncture headache.

4 Outline the management plan for a woman who presents with severe breathlessness in the puerperium.

5 What are the signs and symptoms of a woman who has a uterine infection? Discuss the management.

6 Define secondary postpartum haemorrhage and discuss management of care.

TRUE OR FALSE?

Are the following statements true or false?

7 The most common causative organism for a urinary tract infection is *Escherichia coli*.

8 Pleural effusion may be caused by a venous thromboembolic event.

9 D-dimer is a haematological test commonly used in pregnancy to aid diagnosis of a venous thromboembolic event.

10 Expressing breast milk to completely empty the breasts is a recommended management option for women with mastitis.

11 A third degree tear is defined as 'injury to the perineum involving the anal sphincter complex (external and internal anal sphincters) and anal epithelium'.

MULTIPLE CHOICE

Identify one correct answer for each of the following.

12 Dyspareunia is:

a) difficult or painful micturition

b) menstrual pain

c) difficult or painful coitus

d) severe after pains

13 The Kleihauer test is used to detect:

a) rubella antibodies

b) leucocytes

c) fetal cells

d) rhesus antibodies

14 Thrombo-prophylaxis in the puerperium should be routinely offered to women who experience two of the following:

a) retention of urine

b) instrumental birth

c) antiphospholipid syndrome

d) prolonged labour

15 Women who are non-immune to rubella in the postnatal period:

a) may not receive a rubella immunisation if breastfeeding

b) may infect others for up to 7 days following rubella immunisation due to the nature of a live vaccine

c) should avoid pregnancy for 28 days following rubella immunisation

d) may not be given a rubella vaccine at the same time as any other vaccine

16 Insulin-dependent diabetic women should be advised that:

a) combined oral contraceptives are unsafe in the puerperium

b) there are no known contraindications to oral contraceptives

c) the progesterone only pill is the contraceptive of choice

d) a progesterone releasing intrauterine device is not recommended

ANSWERS

SHORT ANSWER QUESTIONS

1 **Outline the common complications of the puerperium.**

Complications of the puerperium may be minor or have more serious implications for the woman. A puerperal infection may originate in the genital tract; this may be from a genital tract laceration, a perineal tear or an episiotomy site. A urinary tract infection, a breast infection or a wound infection from a caesarean section are other sites that may cause infection. Postpartum haemorrhage, either primary or secondary, may occur. A primary PPH occurs in the first 24 hours following birth and may be defined a minor (500–1,000 ml), major (more than 1000 ml) or severe (more than 2000 ml). A secondary PPH is defined as a prolonged or excessive blood loss from 24 hours after birth and up to 6 weeks postpartum. A deep vein thrombosis or a pulmonary embolism may also occur. Psychological deviations from the normal include third day postnatal 'baby blues', postnatal depression or puerperal psychosis.

2 **Discuss a management plan for a woman who is unable to pass urine postnatally.**

The inability of a woman to pass urine 6 hours following delivery needs attention. However, women who are symptomatic of voiding dysfunction such as slow urinary stream, urinary frequency, incomplete emptying and incontinence also need a management plan. It is important to recognise that acute retention of urine can be painless in the postpartum period especially following epidural analgesia. Urinary retention can be described as either overt when there is an inability to void postpartum or covert when a woman has an elevated residual urine volume of greater than 150 ml following bladder voiding with no symptoms of urinary retention. Management guidelines may differ but the following may be followed and there should be a multidisciplinary approach.

The time and volume of first voiding of the bladder following delivery should be recorded in the woman's postpartum record. If bladder emptying has not occurred within 6 hours of delivery or catheter removal, the woman's bladder should be emptied by catheterisation (in and out) and the volume of urine recorded in the woman's postpartum record. If the volume of urine drained by catheterisation is less than 500 ml, the next voided volume and the postvoid residual (PVR) needs to be measured either by catheterisation (in and out) again or by bladder scan. If the PVR is less than 150 ml, no further action needs to be taken. If the drained volume on the first instance is more than 500 ml or the PVR is more than 150 ml after the second void, an indwelling catheter should be inserted. The catheter should be then left in situ for 24 hours and the medical team consulted.

All women whose initial voided volume is less than 250 ml or report any symptoms of voiding dysfunction should have their postvoid residual volumes measured and then the same protocol as above should be followed.

3 **What is a postdural puncture headache? Briefly outline the midwife's role in caring for a woman who is diagnosed with a postdural puncture headache.**

A postdural puncture occurs when there is an unintentional puncture of the dura with a needle while a woman is undergoing epidural or spinal anaesthesia. Then inadvertent leakage of cerebrospinal fluid occurs from the hole made by the needle. This then reduces the CSF pressure in the spine and leads to a loss of buoyancy supporting the brain and a headache ensues. A postdural puncture headache will usually manifest within 24 hours of the procedure and is typically relieved when the woman lies down. It may sometimes present as a feeling of 'fullness' in the head, dizziness, tinnitus or pain in the neck.

Hydration and analgesia are important factors; women should be encouraged to drink at least 3 litres of fluid daily – if they are unable to do so an intravenous infusion may be necessary.

The midwife should ensure that analgesia is administered at regular intervals; paracetamol and diclofenac sodium are the analgesics of choice. The midwife should facilitate a review by an anaesthetist who will manage the care. Laxatives may be recommended as straining during a bowel movement may make the headache worse. Midwives should also advise women to avoid heavy lifting, again to avoid straining.

The majority of women will need an epidural blood patch performed. This procedure is similar to the original spinal or epidural: under aseptic conditions a needle is inserted into the epidural space and a small amount of maternal blood is injected into the space. The blood will clot and plug the hole in the dura and no further CSF will leak out. Following the procedure the midwife should advise the woman to remain lying down for 2–4 hours and help her to maintain hydration and analgesia. The woman should also be advised not to do any heavy lifting for at least two days. The epidural blood patch should be effective in curing the headache within a few minutes to a few hours in up to 70% of women. A second epidural blood patch may be needed if the headache persists for 24–48 hours following the first epidural blood patch; further epidural blood patches are extremely rare.

4 **Outline the management plan for a woman who presents with severe breathlessness in the puerperium.**

Any signs of breathlessness in the puerperium should be treated with importance. The midwife's priority should be an urgent medical consultation at a consultant obstetric unit. Thromboembolism still remains a leading cause of all direct maternal deaths in the UK. Pregnancy is a risk factor for VTE and is associated with a tenfold increase in risk. Thromboembolic events occur at a rate of 1 in 1000 women during pregnancy and 2 in 1000 women in the puerperium. The prothrombotic changes of pregnancy revert to a pre-pregnancy state at approximately 6 weeks following birth. A pulmonary embolus usually occurs when a thrombus has broken free from a deep vein thrombosis. The site of a DVT may present with swelling and localised redness and tenderness. Signs and symptoms of a pulmonary embolism include chest pain, dyspnoea, tachycardia and haemoptysis. Complications of a pulmonary embolus include cardiac arrest leading to sudden death, pleural effusion, heart failure and arrhythmias. On admission a full history should be taken. Observations of temperature, pulse, blood pressure and respiratory rate should be carried out regularly. Oxygen saturation and arterial blood gases should be performed, O_2 may be administered. A chest X-ray should be performed to exclude other pathology such as fractured ribs, pneumothorax, pneumonia or chest infection. Haematological tests performed are a full blood count (FBC), coagulation screen, urea and electrolytes, and liver function tests. Perfusion scanning is used to confirm diagnosis of a pulmonary embolus. Treatment is by intravenous heparin initially; in the postnatal period women may be offered oral treatment of warfarin after the third day postpartum (or longer if at risk of a PPH). Therapeutic anticoagulant levels should be maintained until 6 weeks postpartum and may be continued for up to 6 months postpartum. It is safe to continue breastfeeding while on heparin or warfarin treatment. The combined oral contraceptive pill is contraindicated following VTE; the progesterone only pill and/or barrier methods should be recommended.

5 **What are the signs and symptoms of a woman who has a uterine infection? Discuss the management.**

Generalised signs and symptoms of an infection include pyrexia, feeling unwell, rigors and tachycardia. Examination of the lochia for amount and odour and palpation of the uterus are needed to ascertain appropriate involution and to assess signs of uterine tenderness. Haematological tests include an FBC to detect a raised white cell count and a CRP may be obtained. A high and/or low vaginal swab and blood cultures may indicate the causative organism and a course of antibiotics will be required to treat the infection. Paracetamol will help to reduce the pyrexia and further analgesia should be considered to help alleviate uterine pain. Midwives should be alert to the possibility that a uterine infection can cause a secondary postpartum haemorrhage.

6   **Define secondary postpartum haemorrhage and discuss management of care.**

A secondary postpartum haemorrhage (PPH) is defined as prolonged or excessive blood loss from 24 hours after birth and up to 6 weeks postpartum; the amount of blood loss has no definition. On occasions the blood loss from a secondary PPH may dictate that management is that of a major obstetric haemorrhage; however the blood loss from a secondary PPH will usually allow management at ward level. A full and accurate history is always needed to determine the likely cause. Estimation of blood loss, palpation of the uterus and a general assessment of maternal condition is needed – temperature, pulse, blood pressure and respiratory rate. Haematological investigations should include an FBC, CRP, group and save and blood cultures if signs of infection exist. A high and/or low vaginal swab is also necessary should signs of infection be present. Treatment of the bleeding may involve a uterotonic if uterine atony is diagnosed, either by intramuscular injection or by intravenous infusion. Appropriate resuscitative measures should be carried out if the haemorrhage is severe. If retained products of conception are visible within the cervical os they may be removed if it is safe to do so. A cautious approach to surgical interventions such as an evacuation of retained products of conception is advised due to the risk of a perforated uterus, with the decision being taken by a senior obstetrician, but this may be necessary if the bleeding either continues or becomes excessive. If the cause is retained products of conception then a conservative approach is appropriate with administration of antibiotics, analgesia and ongoing assessment of maternal condition until improvement is seen.

TRUE OR FALSE?

7 | The most common causative organism for a urinary tract infection is *Escherichia coli*.

8 | Pleural effusion may be caused by a venous thromboembolic event.

9 | D-dimer is a haematological test commonly used in pregnancy to aid diagnosis of a venous thromboembolic event.

D-dimers can be physiologically raised in pregnancy due to changes in the coagulation system and therefore are not useful when diagnosing VTE in pregnant women.

10 | Expressing breast milk to completely empty the breasts is a recommended management option for women with mastitis.

Mastitis should be treated with antibiotics but women should be encouraged to continue breastfeeding their baby.

11 | A third degree tear is defined as 'injury to the perineum involving the anal sphincter complex (external and internal anal sphincters) and anal epithelium'.

A fourth degree tear is defined as 'injury to the perineum involving the anal sphincter complex (external and internal anal sphincters) and anal epithelium', whereas a third degree tear is defined as 'injury to the perineum involving the anal sphincter complex (3a – less than 50% of EAS torn, 3b – more than 50% EAS torn, 3c – both EAS and IAS torn)'.

MULTIPLE CHOICE
Correct answers in bold italics

12 **Dyspareunia is:**

a) difficult or painful micturition   b) menstrual pain   *c) difficult or painful coitus*   d) severe after pains

13 **The Kleihauer test is used to detect:**

a) rubella antibodies   b) leucocytes   *c) fetal cells*   d) rhesus antibodies

14 **Thrombo-prophylaxis in the puerperium should be routinely offered to women who experience two of the following:**

a) retention of urine   b) instrumental birth   *c) antiphospholipid syndrome* *d) prolonged labour*

15 **Women who are non-immune to rubella in the postnatal period:**

a)   may not receive a rubella immunisation if breastfeeding

b)   may infect others for up to 7 days following rubella immunisation due to the nature of a live vaccine

c)   should avoid pregnancy for 28 days following rubella immunisation

d)   may not be given a rubella vaccine at the same time as any other vaccine

16 **Insulin-dependent diabetic women should be advised that:**

a)   combined oral contraceptives are unsafe in the puerperium

b)   there are no known contraindications to oral contraceptives

c)   the progesterone only pill is the contraceptive of choice

d)   a progesterone releasing intrauterine device is not recommended

8 Pharmacology

SHORT ANSWER QUESTIONS

Write short answers to the following.

1 Briefly describe the standards for practice of administration of medicines for midwives.

2 Outline the role of the student midwife in relation to the administration of medicines.

3 List the symptoms of magnesium sulphate toxicity.

4 What are the signs and symptoms of local anaesthetic toxicity?

5 Outline the current legislation related to 'Midwives' Exemptions'. Name six of the more commonly used medicines on the list, including one for neonatal use. What are the exceptions specifically for student midwives regarding administration of medicines on the 'Midwives' Exemptions'?

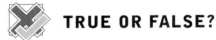

TRUE OR FALSE?

Are the following statements true or false?

6   Syntometrine is the oxytocic drug of choice to accelerate labour.

7   Oral anti-fungals are contraindicated in pregnancy.

8   The recommended dose of folic acid for pre-conceptual women is 5 mcg daily.

9   The half life of a drug is the duration of its action.

10   Oxytocics administered intravenously have a diuretic effect.

11   The M M R vaccine may not be given at the same time as an anti-D immunoglobulin.

12   Low molecular weight heparin is the treatment of choice in pregnancy for V T E as it has a shorter duration of action than unfractionated heparin.

13   Ephedrine is used to correct hypotension by vasodilating blood vessels.

14   Prochlorperazine is used in the treatment of pruritus in pregnancy.

15   Corticosteroids are administered to pregnant women who may be at risk of preterm labour.

MULTIPLE CHOICE

Identify one correct answer for each of the following.

16 Which of the following is NOT a barrier to absorption of a drug:

a) the placenta

b) the gut wall

c) the bronchioles

d) the cell membranes

17 Oxytocin may NOT be administered:

a) orally

b) intravenously

c) into the cord

d) intramuscularly

18 Atosiban is:

a) an oxytocin receptor antagonist

b) an ACE inhibitor

c) an opioid

d) a controlled drug

19 Diclofenac sodium is:

a) a non-steroidal anti-inflammatory drug (NSAID)

b) a cephalosporin

c) an antidiuretic drug

d) an antihypertensive drug

20 Magnesium sulphate is used to treat:

a) hypotension

b) hypoglycaemia

   c) eclamptic seizures

   d) hyperglycaemia

21 Which of the following is a diuretic?

   a) labetalol

   b)   salbutamol

   c) frusemide

   d) glibenclamide

22 Which of the following reduces gastric acid output?

   a) nifedipine

   b) ranitidine

   c) ritodrine

   d) remifentanyl

23 Which of the following is known to be teratogenic in pregnancy?

   a) co-amoxyclav

   b) prochlorperazine

   c) lithium

   d) lorazepam

24 Which of the following is an antihypertensive?

   a) ondansetron

   b) misoprostil

   c) hyoscine

   d) hydralazine

25 Colloids are commonly used:

   a) for treatment of asthma

   b) for treatment of hypocapnia

   c) rectally

   d) for increasing plasma volume

ANSWERS

SHORT ANSWER QUESTIONS

1 | **Briefly describe the standards for practice of administration of medicines for midwives.**

A midwife may administer medicines once she has checked that the product is appropriate for the woman. The midwife must be certain of the identity of the recipient and that the woman is not allergic to the medicine. The midwife must know the therapeutic uses of the medicine and its normal dosage, side effects, precautions and contraindications. The midwife must also know the woman's plan of care, and must check the prescription and label on the medicine is clearly written and unambiguous. The expiry date must be checked, and consideration must be given to the dosage, weight (where appropriate) as well as the method of administration, route and timing of the medicine. Administration of a medicine must be given in context to the woman's condition. The midwife must contact either the prescriber or another prescriber should any of the following occur: contraindications to the prescribed medicine as discovered; the woman develops a reaction to the medicine; or where assessment of the woman indicates that the medicine is no longer suitable. Midwives should also make a clear, accurate and immediate record of all medicines administered, intentionally withheld or refused by a woman; the signature should be clear and legible. It is also the midwife's responsibility to record when delegation of administration is made to another professional.

2 | **Outline the role of the student midwife in relation to the administration of medicines.**

The student midwife is regulated by the Nursing and Midwifery Council (NMC) and must comply with all rules, standards, guidance and advice. Standard 17 of the *Standards for Pre-registration Midwifery Education* (NMC 2009) state that 'students must be able at the point of registration to select, acquire and administer safely a range of permitted drugs consistent with legislation, applying knowledge and skills to the situation which pertains at the time. Methods of administration include: oral, intravenous, intramuscular, topical and inhalational'. The NMC allows student midwives to administer medicines on the midwives' exemptions list, except controlled drugs or PGDs, under the direct supervision of a midwife who must be a sign off mentor.

Direct means 'in visual contact during which time the midwife observes the act of administration of medicines by a student midwife' (NMC Circular 07/2011 p. 3). Student midwives may not administer controlled drugs or PGDs. They may, however, participate in the checking and preparation of medicines for administration on the midwives' exemptions list and PoMs under the direct supervision of a sign off mentor (NMC 2011).

3 List the symptoms of magnesium sulphate toxicity.

Magnesium sulphate is used to treat convulsions arising from eclampsia and to prevent further convulsions. The symptoms of magnesium toxicity include loss of patellar reflexes, weakness, nausea, sensation of warmth, flushing, drowsiness, double vision and slurred speech, respiratory depression, arrhythmias and cardiac arrest. Calcium gluconate injection is used to treat magnesium toxicity.

4 What are the signs and symptoms of local anaesthetic toxicity?

Local anaesthetic toxicity occurs when a local anaesthetic enters the systemic circulation, for example following the siting of an epidural. Symptoms include numbness of the tongue or lips, tinnitus, light-headedness and anxiety or a feeling of foreboding. Signs include slurring of the speech, drowsiness, convulsions and cardio-respiratory arrest.

5 Outline the current legislation related to 'Midwives' Exemptions'. Name six of the more commonly used medicines on the list, including one for neonatal use. What are the exceptions specifically for student midwives regarding administration of medicines on the 'Midwives' Exemptions'?

Midwives can supply and administer for non-parenteral use prescription only from a list of 25 medicines. Commonly used ones include: oral diclofenac, oral phytomenadione (for neonatal use), IM anti-D immunoglobulin, IM cyclizine lactate, IM diamorphine, IV Hartmann's solution, IM/IV oxytocics, IM naloxone (for neonatal use).

Student midwives may not administer controlled drugs or PGDs. They may, however, observe the activity.

TRUE OR FALSE?

6 **Syntometrine is the oxytocic drug of choice to accelerate labour.**

Syntometrine can be used in active management of third stage of labour or for a PPH. It consists of 0.5 mg of ergometrine and 5 units of syntocinon in 1 ml.

7 **Oral anti-fungals are contraindicated in pregnancy.**

Oral anti-fungals are contraindicated in pregnancy, but some anti-fungals are safe to use in pregnancy by vaginal application such as clotrimazole.

8 **The recommended dose of folic acid for pre-conceptual women is 5 mcg daily.**

The recommended dose of folic acid for pre-conceptual woman is 400 mcg daily up to 12 weeks of pregnancy.

9 **The half life of a drug is the duration of its action.**

The half life of a drug is the time taken for the concentration of the drug in the blood or plasma to fall to half its maximum value.

10 **Syntocinon has a diuretic effect.**

Syntocinon causes retention of water in the body.

11 **The MMR vaccine may not be given at the same time as an anti-D immunoglobulin.**

The MMR vaccine is administered in the postnatal period and can be given at the same time as anti-D immunoglobulin. Administration must be using separate syringes and given into two different limbs.

12 **Low molecular weight heparin is the treatment of choice in pregnancy for VTE as it has a shorter duration of action than unfractionated heparin.**

LMWH is the treatment of choice for VTE in pregnancy because it has a longer duration of action than unfractionated heparin therefore it has a more predictable dose response, which allows for a once daily administration. It also has a reduced incidence of side effects.

13 **Ephedrine is used to correct hypotension by vasodilating blood vessels.**

Ephedrine is used to correct hypotension by constricting the peripheral vessels. Its use in obstetrics is to reverse hypotension associated with epidural and spinal anaesthesia.

14 **Prochlorperazine is used in the treatment of pruritus in pregnancy.**

Prochlorperazine is an antiemetic and is used for the treatment of nausea and vomiting in pregnancy.

15 **Corticosteroids are administered to pregnant women who may be at risk of preterm labour.**

Corticosteroids help reduce the risk of respiratory distress syndrome in preterm infants by enhancing the production of surfactant in the fetus.

MULTIPLE CHOICE
Correct answers in bold italics

16 **Which of the following is NOT a barrier to absorption of a drug:**

a) the placenta   b) the gut wall   c) the bronchioles   *d) the cell membranes*

17 **Oxytocin may NOT be administered:**

a) orally   b) intravenously   c) into the cord   d) intramuscularly

18 **Atosiban is:**

a) an oxytocin receptor antagonist   b) an ACE inhibitor   c) an opioid
d) a controlled drug

19 **Diclofenac sodium is:**

a) a non-steroidal anti-inflammatory drug (NSAID)   b) a cephalosporin
c) an antidiurestic drug   d) an antihypertensive drug

20 **Magnesium sulphate is used to treat:**

a) hypotension   b) hypoglycaemia   *c) eclamptic seizures*   d) hyperglycaemia

21 **Which of the following is a diuretic?**

a) labetalol   b) salbutamol   *c) frusemide*   d) glibenclamide

22 **Which of the following reduces gastric acid output?**

a) nifedipine   *b) ranitidine*   c) ritodrine   d) remifentanyl

23 **Which of the following is known to be teratogenic in pregnancy?**

a) co-amoxyclav   b) prochlorperazine   *c) lithium*   d) lorazepam

24 **Which of the following is an antihypertensive?**

a) ondansetron   b) misoprostil   c) hyoscine   *d)   hydralazine*

25 **Colloids are commonly used:**

a) for treatment of asthma   b) for treatment of hypocapnia   c) rectally
d) for increasing plasma volume

9 Numeracy

In this chapter you will find a series of questions that will help you to assess your ability to carry out simple calculations in midwifery practice. First, however, there is a brief guide to performing a number of common types of calculation.

GUIDE TO CALCULATION

The following formulae are a guide to some of the common numerical calculations a midwife will need to make in the clinical area. A basic level of mathematical knowledge is assumed.

1 SI units

The metric or SI system is used in healthcare. When converting to either a higher or lower unit multiply or divide by 1000.

For example:

Larger unit	Smaller unit
1 metre	1000 millimetres (length)
1 litre	1000 millilitres (capacity or volume)
1 gram	1000 milligrams (mg) (weight or mass)
1 milligram	1000 micrograms (mcg)
1 mole	1000 millimoles (mmol) (mass of molecules)

2 Percentages

Per cent means 'out of a hundred' and can be written as a fraction.
For example: 20/100 can be simplified to 2/10.

To calculate one number as a percentage of another number:

First write the percentage required as a fraction.
Then multiply that fraction by the other number.

For example: 15% of 180

$$\frac{15 \times 180}{100} = 27$$

3 Proportions

It may be necessary to calculate a proportion of a drug required, either reconstituted injections or syrups.

The formula is:

$$\text{Amount required} = \frac{\text{amount prescribed} \times \text{volume of fluid}}{\text{amount in each measure}}$$

OR

$$\text{Dose that you want} = \frac{\text{what you need} \times \text{volume that you have}}{\text{what you have got}}$$

For example: amoxycillin 125 mg is prescribed and is available in 500 mg vials, to be reconstituted in 10 ml of water for injections.

$$\frac{\text{Dose you want is 125 mg} \times \text{volume of 10 ml}}{\text{the dose you have is 500 mg}} = 2.5 \text{ ml}$$

4 Infant feeding

You may need to calculate the amount of feed required for a baby based on volume of milk required per kilogram of body weight and number of feeds in a 24 hour period.

The formula is therefore:

$$\frac{\text{Actual weight of baby (kg)} \times \text{ml per kg}}{\text{Number of feeds in 24 hours}}$$

For example: a 3 kg baby needs 120 ml of milk per kilo per 24 hour period and is being fed 3 hourly.

$$\frac{3 \times 120}{8} = 45 \text{ ml per feed}$$

5 Calculating body mass index

The formula for calculating a BMI is:

$$\frac{\text{Weight (kg)}}{\text{Height (m)}^2}$$

First multiply the height measurement by itself (height squared).
Then take the weight and divide it by the figure of the height squared.
For example: a 1.68 m woman who weighs 88 kg.
$1.68 \times 1.68 = 2.82$
$88 \div 2.82 = 31.20$
Rounded to the nearest whole number BMI = 31

6 Calculation of intravenous infusion rates

An IVI is calculated by drops per minute. Differing types of infusion sets and differing types of viscosity and fluids will influence the drop rate. Infusion sets may vary their drop rate by 10–60 drops per minute.

The formula for calculating an infusion rate is:

$$\frac{\text{Drops per ml (of giving set)} \times \text{total amount of infusion (ml)}}{\text{Time of infusion in minutes}}$$

For example:
A woman needs 500 ml of normal saline over 6 hours using a 15 ml drops/min giving set.

$$\frac{15 \text{ (drop rate)} \times 500 \text{ (volume to be infused)}}{360 \text{ minutes (6 hours} \times 60 \text{ mins)}} \qquad \frac{15 \times 500}{360} = 20.83$$

If a decimal is the result then the number must be rounded up or down as drops per minute can only be given as a whole number, therefore **21 ml per minute** should be administered.

7 Converting fractions to decimals

Fractions are written as one number over another number i.e. ½ (one half)
Decimals are expressed as a number to the right of a decimal point and express tenths, hundredths, thousandths etc. depending on how far to the right of the decimal point the number extends i.e. 2.55.

To convert fractions to a decimal divide the top number of the fraction by the bottom number.

For example:

7/20   7 divided by 20 = 0.35

NUMERACY QUESTIONS

1   A baby weighs 4200 grams, convert this weight to kilograms.

2   Which is larger, 0.3 or 0.03 litres?

3   Convert 0.5 g to mg.

4   How many grams in a kilogram?

5   Change 3/8 to a decimal, correct to one decimal place.

6   Convert 250 mg to g.

7   A baby weighs 3.25 kg, convert this to grams.

8   A woman receives three doses of paracetamol 1 g. How many milligrams has she received?

9   Convert 250 mcg to mg.

10   A linctus is available as 10 mg/ml; the prescription is for 20 mg, how many ml will be given?

11   You are required to give dexamethasone 12 mg from a supply of 4 mg/ml ampoule. What amount should be drawn up?

12   Syntometrine contains 0.5 mg ergometrine. Express this as micrograms.

13 An 1800 g preterm baby requires 60 ml/kg milk in the first 24 hours. The baby will be fed 2 hourly. Calculate the amount of milk required for each feed.

14 Following a difficult birth, a 3 kg baby is prescribed neonatal paracetamol suspension. The dose is 10 mg/kg. Paracetamol suspension is 120 mg in 5 ml. What volume of neonatal paracetamol suspension will be given?

15 A baby weighs 3.8 kg at birth. Four days later it has lost 10% of its birth weight. How much does it weigh now?

16 A woman has been prescribed 600 mg of clindamycin. The stock dose is 150 mg/ml. How many ml are required?

17 One unit of whole blood is to be infused over 3 hours, the volume to be infused is 350 ml. The giving set infuses at 15 drops per ml. Calculate the infusion rate per minute, giving the answer to the nearest ml.

18 1000 ml of normal saline is to be administered over 6 hours; if 20 drops equals 1 ml, how many drops per minute should be administered. Give the answer to the nearest whole number.

19 Body mass index is calculated by weight in kilograms divided by height in metres squared. A woman weighs 98 kg and is 1.75 m tall. What is her BMI?

20 A baby weighing 3.6 kg is to receive ampicillin intravenously. The dose required is 25 mg per kg body weight per 24 hours. How much should the baby receive per dose if the ampicillin is prescribed 8 hourly?

21 A woman is allowed to have 30 ml fluid per hour per kg of body weight and weighs 84 kg. How much fluid may she have in a 6 hour period?

22 Amoxicillin syrup is available as 125 mg/ml. Calculate the volume required for 375 mg.

23 An infusion of 100 units of Actrapid insulin is made up to a volume of 100 ml with normal saline. How many units of insulin per ml does this equal?

24 An ampoule of neonatal naloxone hydrochloride contains 2 ml of naloxone, with 20 microgams per ml. The usual dose of naloxone is 10 micrograms per kilo. How many ml is needed to give to a 3 kg baby?

25 The average blood volume for a non-pregnant woman is 5 litres. In pregnancy the blood volume increases by 40%. Calculate the blood volume in a pregnant woman.

26 A student midwife works two 12-hour shifts and has three study days of 6.5 hours each. How many hours has she undertaken this week?

27 Calculate the total fluid balance for this woman:

Input		
I V Oral		
350 ml	450 ml	
Output		
Urine	Vomit	Drain
150 ml	100 ml	50 ml

28 Three tablets each contain 250 mg, what is the total dose in milligrams?

29 The prescription is for 625 mg, the tablet dose is 1.25 g each. How many tablets will be given?

30 If a woman needs 1000 ml saline over 12 hours with a drop rate of 15 per ml, what is the flow rate of the infusion per minute (give the answer to the nearest whole number)?

ANSWERS TO NUMERACY QUESTIONS

1   A baby weighs 4200 grams, convert this weight to kilograms. 4.2 kg

2   Which is larger, 0.3 or 0.03 litres? 0.3 litres

3   Convert 0.5 g to mg. 500 mg

4   How many grams in a kilogram? 1000 g

5   Change 3/8 to a decimal, correct to one decimal place. 0.4

6   Convert 250 mg to g. 0.25 g

7   A baby weighs 3.25 kg, convert this to grams. 3250 g

8   A woman receives three doses of paracetamol 1 g. How many milligrams has she received? 3000 mg

9   Convert 250 mcg to mg. 0.25 mg

10   A linctus is available as 10 mg/ml; the prescription is for 20 mg, how many ml will be given? 2 ml

11   You are required to give dexamethasone 12 mg from a supply of 4 mg/ml ampoule. What amount should be drawn up? 3 ml

12   Syntometrine contains 0.5 mg ergometrine. Express this as micrograms. 500 mcg

13 An 1800 g preterm baby requires 60 ml/kg milk in the first 24 hours. The baby will be fed 2 hourly. Calculate the amount of milk required for each feed. 9 ml

14 Following a difficult birth, a 3 kg baby is prescribed neonatal paracetamol suspension. The dose is 10 mg/Kg. Paracetamol suspension is 120 mg in 5 ml. What volume of neonatal paracetamol suspension will be given? 1.25 ml

15 A baby weighs 3.8 kg at birth. Four days later it has lost 10% of its birth weight. How much does it weigh now? 3.42 kg

16 A woman has been prescribed 600 mg of clindamycin. The stock dose is 150 mg/ml. How many ml are required? 4 ml

17 One unit of whole blood is to be infused over 3 hours, the volume to be infused is 350 ml. The giving set infuses at 15 drops per ml. Calculate the infusion rate per minute, giving the answer to the nearest ml. 29 drops per minute

18 1000 ml of normal saline is to be administered over 6 hours, if 20 drops equals 1 ml, how many drops per minute should be administered. Give the answer to the nearest whole number. 56 drops per minute

19 Body mass index is calculated by weight in kilograms divided by height in metres squared. A woman weighs 98 kg and is 1.75 m tall. What is her BMI? 32

20 A baby weighing 3.6 kg is to receive ampicillin intravenously. The dose required is 25 mg per kg body weight per 24 hours. How much should the baby receive per dose if the ampicillin is prescribed 8 hourly? 30 mg

21 A woman is allowed to have 30 ml fluid per 24 hours per kilogram of body weight and weighs 84 kg. How much fluid may she have in a 6 hour period? 630 ml

22 Amoxicillin syrup is available as 125 mg/ml. Calculate the volume required for 375 mg. 3 ml

23 An infusion of 100 units of Actrapid insulin is made up to a volume of 100 ml with normal saline. How many units of insulin per ml does this equal? 1 unit

24 An ampoule of neonatal naloxone hydrochloride contains 2 ml of naloxone, with 20 microgams per ml. The usual dose of naloxone is 10 micrograms per kilo. How many ml is needed to give to a 3 kg baby? 1.5 ml

25 The average blood volume for a non-pregnant woman is 5 litres. In pregnancy the blood volume increases by 40%. Calculate the blood volume in a pregnant woman. 7 litres

26 A student midwife works two 12-hour shifts and has two study days of 6.5 hours each. How many hours has she undertaken this week? 37 hours

27 Calculate the total fluid balance for this woman:

Input		
I V Oral		
350 ml	450 ml	
Output		
Urine	Vomit	Drain
150 ml	100 ml	50 ml

500 ml positive balance

28 Three tablets each contain 250 mg. What is the total dose in milligrams? 750 mg

29 The prescription is for 625 mg, the tablet dose is 1.25 g each. How many tablets will be given? One half tablet

30 If a woman needs 1000 ml saline over 12 hours with a drop rate of 15 per ml, what is the flow rate of the infusion per minute (give the answer to the nearest whole number)? 21 drops per minute

Glossary

Alkalaemia: increased alkalinity of the blood

Capacitation: a process whereby the sperm are conditioned whilst in the female reproductive tract en route to fertilising the ovum

Chloasma: skin pigmentation seen in pregnancy on the forehead, nose and cheeks

Cricoid pressure: backward pressure on the cricoid cartilage to occlude the oesophagus

D Dimers: a blood test that detects the fibrin degredation product known as 'D dimer', seen in the blood following degradation of a blood clot

Endocytosis: process of cellular ingestion whereby a cell takes in outside materials by engulfing them with its plasma membrane

Epididymis: a coiled structure providing storage and transport of spermatozoa

Erythrocyte: red blood cell

Erythropoeisis: formation of red blood cells

Expiratory reserve volume: the additional volume of air expired after a normal expiration

Ferguson's reflex: a positive feedback response to pressure on the cervix

Haemodilution: increase of plasma in the blood

Hyperbilirubinaemia: excessive levels of bilirubin in the blood

Hyperemesis: excessive vomiting

Hypocapnia: reduced carbon dioxide levels in the blood

LAM: lactational amenorrhoea method, a method of natural family planning

Lanugo: fine hair covering the fetus in utero

Meiosis: cell division resulting in a gamete that has half the amount of chromosomes present, in preparation for sexual reproduction

Nephron: the functioning unit of a kidney

Oogenesis: formation and production of an ovum

Perimetrium: a layer of peritoneum that covers the uterovesical pouch and the pouch of Douglas

Pica: cravings for non-nutritive substances

Pinocytosis: a process whereby a cell ingests extracellular fluids

Striae gravidarum: skin marks caused by stretching

Syncope: fainting

Tidal volume: the volume of air inspired or expired in a single breath

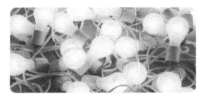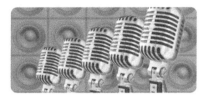
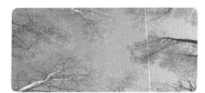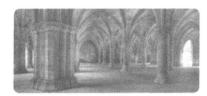
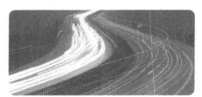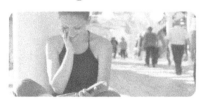
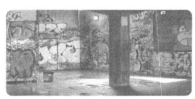